Multiple Sclerosis

D0161924

A Tavistock Professional Book

The Experience of Illness
Series Editors: Ray Fitzpatrick and Stanton Newman

Multiple Sclerosis

Ian Robinson

Routledge

First published in 1988 by Routledge
11 New Fetter Lane, London EC4P 4EE

© 1988 Ian Robinson

Typeset in 10/12pt Times, Linotron 202
by Input Typesetting, London SW19
Printed in Great Britain
by Richard Clay Ltd, Bungay, Suffolk

All rights reserved. No part of this book may be
reprinted or reproduced or utilized in any form or
by any electronic, mechanical, or other means, now
known or hereafter invented, including photocopying
and recording, or in any information storage or
retrieval system, without permission in writing from
the publishers.

British Library Cataloguing in Publication Data

Robinson, Ian, *1943–*
  Multiple sclerosis.—(The experience of illness series).
  1. Man. Multiple sclerosis. Personal adjustment
  I. Title II. Series
  362.1'96834

ISBN 0–415–60634–1
ISBN 0–415–00635–X Pbk

Contents

Editors' preface vii

Preface ix

1 Understanding multiple sclerosis 1

2 Solving the puzzle: from the onset of symptoms to the diagnosis of multiple sclerosis 14

3 Life with multiple sclerosis: subjective experience and the disease 29

4 Life with multiple sclerosis: social context and consequences 50

5 The experience of managing multiple sclerosis 78

6 Sources of support: possibilities and problems 101

7 Making sense of the future: maintaining faith and hope 125

References 138

Index 147

Editors' preface

The aim of this series is to integrate the personal accounts of individuals who experience illness with the growing sociological and psychological literature. Ian Robinson vividly portrays the reality of multiple sclerosis by drawing on a rich body of research material.

Individuals with multiple sclerosis describe the lengthy and often distressing phase prior to the formal diagnosis. Varying symptoms remain unexplained and when eventually contact is made with the doctor the continuing uncertainty often leads to further frustration. The course of multiple sclerosis varies considerably from one individual to another and the future for any individual is often unpredictable. The uncertainty that this evokes is graphically conveyed by the author. Patients respond with a variety of coping strategies, the complexity of which is well illustrated.

A further issue that individuals have to contend with is the absence of any treatment of established efficacy. This throws individuals on to their own resources and impels them to seek other forms of accommodation and solutions. The courage and hope that some individuals are able to bring to bear illustrate some of the positive themes Ian Robinson has found in patients' accounts.

The book also examines how disability may lead to dependence on others and how voluntary and self-help groups can provide a powerful sense of identity and control over the illness. Ian Robinson examines the debates on the contribution such organizations make in this area.

Those who look to the social sciences to illuminate and inform ideas about health and illness will find in this volume a revealing and moving analysis of one major illness.

Preface

The main source on which this book is based is a collection of over 400 life stories of people with multiple sclerosis and members of their families from Australia, Canada, and the USA as well as the United Kingdom. The life stories have provided invaluable insights into how people manage life with multiple sclerosis, and richly supplement other evidence about the meaning, impact, and experience of living with the disease. In the book all names of individuals have been changed to preserve confidentiality, as has other information which might identify those concerned.

The life stories form part of a large collection of quantitative and qualitative information on the epidemiological, personal, and social aspects of multiple sclerosis which is held at Brunel, the University of West London. It is at this university that a research unit into these aspects of the disease has been established and funded by Action for Research into Multiple Sclerosis (ARMS). The initiative of the Chief Executive of ARMS, John Simkins, which resulted in the founding of the unit, and the continuing support of ARMS and its members for its research projects, is gratefully acknowledged.

I would also particularly like to acknowledge the support and encouragement of Judith Monks and Anna Wynne, as well as for their careful reading of an earlier version of the text, from which I have benefited considerably. I owe a debt of gratitude to many others, especially Julia Segal, on whose knowledge and experience I have drawn. Jenny Charteris has been of immense administrative help in organizing the preparation of the manuscript. The editors of this series have exercised a patient and facilitating role which has expedited the completion of this book. For my wife Jane and son Alistair the preparation of the manuscript has involved considerable sacrifices and I thank them for their forbearance.

Finally I would like to express gratitude to the many people with multiple sclerosis, and members of their families, who have been prepared to contribute to this research. In a real sense without their contributions this book could not have been written. I hope that they will feel that I have done justice to their personal accounts and will feel that they have enabled others to learn from their experiences.

Chapter one

Understanding multiple sclerosis

Multiple sclerosis is a disease of unknown aetiology, variable onset, problematic diagnosis, unpredictable prognosis, and no effective treatment. Many features of the disease are therefore the subject of intense speculation and controversy. The debate about the nature of multiple sclerosis conditions its clinical diagnosis and management, as well as research into all aspects of the disease. The experience of people with multiple sclerosis is thus mediated not only through the uncertainties, problems, and difficulties of their personal and social world, but also through the spectrum of medical uncertainty and dispute about key aspects of the disease. In this chapter there is an introductory discussion of some of these uncertainties and disputes.

Describing multiple sclerosis

One of the standard definitions of the disease is provided by Walton, who describes it as

A disease of unknown aetiology characterised pathologically by the widespread occurrence in the nervous system of patches of demyelination followed by gliosis. In many cases the early manifestations of the disease are followed by conspicuous improvement, so that remissions and relapses are a striking feature of the disorder, the course of which may be thus prolonged for many years. The early symptoms are often those of focal lesions of the central nervous system, while the later clinical picture is one of progressive dissemination tending to produce the classic features of ataxic paraplegia.

(Walton 1977: 544)

1

This definition is a succinct medical description of multiple sclerosis, and it also indicates the likely variability and uncertainty in relation to the condition. From a patient's point of view such a description may understate the range and nature of the symptoms and experiences to which the disease may give rise, in its early as well as its later stages. The experience of the onset of the disease is more fully considered in Chapter 2, but it is important to indicate that both the clinical and personal interpretation of the initial symptoms can be at variance with the subsequent diagnosis of multiple sclerosis.

A more graphic indication of the variability of the disease is given in this further description by Schumacher and his colleagues.

> Multiple sclerosis is a disorder characterised in cross-section by symptoms and signs of neurologic dysfunction indicating multiple and separate lesions in the central nervous system. Symptoms appear longitudinally in the form of acutely or slowly developing episodes scattered over a period of time. Individual attacks may assume a variety of patterns. The overall course is made up of multiple attacks or of erratic or steady progression over prolonged periods, usually many years. . . . Regardless of the course assumed by an attack, subsequent recurrence or steady progression usually leads ultimately to chronic and permanent disability.
>
> (Schumacher *et al*. 1965: 553)

This account of multiple sclerosis emphasizes both the symptomatic variation and the different courses that the disease may take.

Diagnosing multiple sclerosis

The diagnosis, assessment, and classification of multiple sclerosis is undertaken on the basis of clinical examinations supported by an increasing range of technical investigations. The role of these investigations in the diagnosis of the disease is a matter of continuing debate. In a condition as complex as multiple sclerosis, where reported or observable symptoms may be at variance with the results of laboratory tests – or such tests themselves may be indeterminate – the overriding importance of clinical judgement has been emphasized (Poser 1984: 233). In this context the status of the formal neurological examination, following established diagnostic criteria, remains of paramount significance.

A neurological examination for multiple sclerosis involves a consideration of current signs and symptoms, as well as an investigation of the clinical history. One of the problems in making a definitive diagnosis of the disease is that many of the early symptoms can individually or severally be as indicative of other conditions as they can be of multiple sclerosis. In order to make a distinction between cases of the disease with an established diagnosis, and those in which the diagnosis is unclear, or provisional, McAlpine, Lumsden, and Acheson (1972) proposed three diagnostic categories – definite, probable, and possible. These three categories have come to be widely accepted as a basis on which assessments of potential cases of multiple sclerosis are considered.

For the category 'definite' multiple sclerosis a variety of diagnostic criteria have been used in the assessment of the disease. One of the most widely deployed has been that of Schumacher *et al.* (1965). According to these criteria there must be

1 evidence of objective neurological abnormality
2 evidence of involvement of two or more separate parts of the central nervous system (CNS)
3 a predominant white matter basis to the CNS disease
4 slow progression of signs and symptoms, or two or more exacerbations separated by at least one month
5 an age range of 10 to 50 inclusive at the onset of symptoms
6 no better alternative explanation by a clinical neurologist.

These criteria were constructed before the advent of a number of additional laboratory techniques, which have now become available. None the less the clinically oriented approach of Schumacher and his colleagues has come to be accepted even in more recent criteria (Poser *et al.* 1983). As both sets of criteria indicate, a combination of signs and symptoms characterize the disease, a number of which may become apparent only through observation over time. In an attempt to foreshorten diagnostic uncertainty, and to provide definitive evidence as to its existence in an individual, the pathology of the disease has been intensively studied. Some components of the pathological jigsaw of the disease are well established, although the clinical manifestation of these pathological signs may be subject to considerable variation.

The pathology of multiple sclerosis – reading the signs

An apparently typical pathological feature of multiple sclerosis is the existence of sclerotic plaques or lesions mainly in the white matter of the brain and spinal cord – from which the name of the disease derives. These plaques are caused by the demyelination of nerve fibres. The exact size, nature, and location of the sclerotic plaques is now open to more precise determination with the development of techniques such as computerized tomography (CT) and more recently nuclear magnetic resonance (NMR) imaging. These imaging techniques are beginning to reveal information which may call into question existing assumptions about the nature of the disease. In particular patients with single symptoms, on whom imaging has been undertaken at an apparently early stage of their disease, reveal the presence of multiple lesions – without corresponding clinical symptoms (Ormerod *et al.* 1986; Miller *et al.* 1987). This finding may suggest that the clinical diagnosis of the disease, as being based on disseminations occurring over time with associated clinically observable symptoms, needs reconsideration. So-called 'silent plaques' may have no clearly identified symptomatic effects, and even other actively changing lesions may have no demonstrable symptoms associated with them. At one extreme is the situation where multiple sclerosis has been diagnosed after death in apparently asymptomatic cases, through the existence of lesions on pathological examination (Gilbert and Sadler 1983).

Other pathological signs used to assess the presence of the disease may be subject to equally problematic interpretation. Since the discovery of abnormalities in the cerebro-spinal fluid (CSF) of those with multiple sclerosis, an examination of CSF for indicative oligoclonal bands and other features has become a common procedure. However there are clinically confirmed cases of the disease where these features are not present, and other conditions which may exhibit virtually identical CSF changes.

The involvement of optical symptoms in many cases of multiple sclerosis has led to particular concern with the detection and measurement of the pathology of the optic nerve. Optic neuritis and its consequences, traditionally associated with multiple sclerosis and a number of other conditions, have, until fairly recently, been detected through general clinical examination of the eye. However the difficulty of consistently identifying all cases where optical involvement was suspected has led to the development of new procedures. Perhaps the most widely used techniques in connection with the diagnosis of multiple sclerosis are currently tests of visually evoked potentials (VEP). These tests measure the electrical conductivity of the visual system of the brain, and have been found to produce values for most cases with multiple sclerosis which differ significantly from those of the normal population. The reliability of VEPs as a convincing indicator of multiple sclerosis has been questioned by some, who have argued that a variety of conditions and circumstances may produce values which mimic those found with the disease (Poser 1984: 243). However, for many clinicians VEPs remain the most useful of the generally available diagnostic aids.

Other pathological work has concentrated on immunological aspects of multiple sclerosis, and the detection of abnormal elements in the blood chemistry of people with the disease. It is likely to be some time before tests based on this research are widely deployed to aid diagnosis in clinical practice.

In summary there are continuing developments in the detection and measurement of pathological aspects of multiple sclerosis, particularly relating to those areas which may aid early diagnosis. However a definitive diagnostic indicator of the disease has yet to be found. With such a wide variety of pathological signs, some of which may prove to be apparently contradictory, and others of which may prove to have little or no direct association with observable symptoms, the importance of an overall clinical assessment of the status of an individual case is emphasized. The interpretation of individual symptoms over time, in conjunction with measurement of signs, is particularly important.

Interpreting symptoms in multiple sclerosis

Diagnostic criteria employed in the assessment of multiple sclerosis, such as those of Schumacher *et al.*, emphasize the importance of clinically investigating both signs and symptoms. If the examination of signs is an art – supported by a variety of tests – the interpretation of symptoms in the disease is even more dependent on clinical skill and judgement. The patterning of symptoms, particularly over time, is a crucial component of the diagnosis.

Given the requirement in certain diagnostic criteria for the existence of symptoms in a particular temporal pattern, it can be seen that a definite diagnosis of the disease may not be made at a first medical assessment. Thus a patient seeking medical advice for the first time with visual symptoms, or with disorders of sensation or muscular weakness – all common initial symptoms associated with multiple sclerosis (Matthews *et al.* 1985) – may receive no indication of the possible diagnosis of the disease at that stage. It is the persistence or recurrence of symptoms, as much as their presence at any one time, which is a determining factor in focusing on multiple sclerosis as a potential diagnosis.

The course of and prognosis for multiple sclerosis

The variability of the course of multiple sclerosis is one of its key characteristics. With the possibility of the distinctive lesions of multiple sclerosis occurring at many points in the central nervous system in a relatively unpredictable way, the appearance of the effects of the disease and their timing is particularly problematic to anticipate. Thus a clear and reliable indication as to how the disease will progress in any one case is difficult to achieve. The course of multiple sclerosis may vary from being relatively or completely benign throughout life, to being rapidly progressive and leading to death within a period of months – although it should be noted that this speedy and fatal variant of the disease is statistically rare.

Despite problems associated with the assessment of the course of multiple sclerosis, there are classifications of different temporal patterns of the disease. In an attempt to provide a clinical and research guide to the most common courses that the disease takes, a twofold classification is often employed. Cases may thus be divided into those whose course is progressive, and those whose course is characterized by relapses and remissions.

In summary the course and prognosis of the disease is still a question of debate. There are a number of factors which appear to act as partial prognostic indicators. However even the most significant of these falls far short of indicating decisively how the general course of the disease develops, let alone providing clear guidance in any individual case (Compston 1987b). Further research thus continues to attempt to elucidate the complex course of the disease.

The distribution of multiple sclerosis

Multiple sclerosis is characterized by a particular demographic and geographic distribution. This distribution has assumed a very considerable importance in attempts to understand the disease. In the absence of any clear and agreed view as to the cause of multiple sclerosis, the clues provided by this epidemiological evidence have been used to explore a number of the theories discussed in the next section.

Perhaps the most striking feature of the geographical distribution of multiple sclerosis is high correlation of the prevalence of the disease with temperate latitudes. In Kurtzke's comprehensive review (1980) of all the population prevalence studies up to 1979, the highest prevalence rates are in the latitudes 43° to 65° north in Europe; 37° to 52° north in the Americas; and 34° to 44° south in Australasia. Moderate then low frequency prevalence rates occur both north and south of these latitudes as the Poles and the Equator are approached. The difference between high and low prevalence rates is substantial. In the high prevalence latitudes rates range from 30 to over 80 per 100,000 and in the moderate frequency latitudes from 5 to 25 per 100,000 (Kurtzke 1980: 63–7). There are even lower prevalence rates for other latitudes. However, as the medical and particularly the neurological services in a number of the countries concerned in these very low prevalence areas are relatively undeveloped, some caution must be exercised in interpreting the findings. None the less the pattern of geographical distribution of multiple sclerosis is sufficiently consistent and uniform to warrant special consideration in research to understand the disease.

Another demographic feature of the prevalence of multiple sclerosis, not unrelated to geographical distribution of the disease, has been the finding that populations, other than those which are caucasian in origin, have a lower prevalence rate. This finding has prompted a number of studies related to the possibility of increased or decreased risk of the disease following immigration to high or low prevalence areas. Although such studies are methodologically difficult to undertake, the general finding has been that immigrants tend to retain much of the risk of their birthplace. Other surveys have indicated that immigration before the age of 15 tends to result in the acquisition of the risk of the area to which the immigrant has moved (Alter, Leibowitz, and

7

Speer 1966). However, there must be extreme caution used in interpreting these findings for the relevant factors are extremely complex to identify, research, and evaluate.

Other aspects of the demographic distribution of multiple sclerosis are as interesting and important as its geographical distribution. The age of onset, as indicated in many clinical studies, is predominantly between the ages of 20 and 50, although there are both earlier and later recorded cases. However, it must be remembered that the exact age of onset is often difficult to determine, particularly in those cases where symptoms have materialized in an insidious way. A further feature of the disease is that it affects more women than men. A review of some fifty studies which considered the ratio of women to men with multiple sclerosis found that the ratio was, on average, three women to two men with the diagnosed condition (I. Robinson, Bakes, and Lawson 1983). Wide geographical variations in the sex ratio were uncovered by the studies, whose basis and methodological quality varied substantially.

The cause of multiple sclerosis

The cause of multiple sclerosis is unknown despite the investment of very considerable scientific and other resources in the quest for a definitive aetiology. In this situation a number of theories have gained currency amongst the scientific, medical, and lay communities, although all remain unproven.

One of the critical starting-points for the search for a cause for multiple sclerosis has been the evaluation of the reasons for the concentration of known cases of multiple sclerosis in the temperate latitudes. Mayer correlated both socal and physical factors with the areas of high prevalence of the disease (1981). Climatic and geographical factors such as latitude, hours of sunshine, and mean annual temperature were highly correlated with the prevalence rate, as were a series of factors related to the social and economic development of the areas concerned (Mayer 1981: 261). Others have explored the geographical relationship of the disease with nutrition and diet, as well as with the distribution of domestic and farm animals, following the discovery of the similarity of certain diseases of those animals to multiple sclerosis.

Leading from these broad correlations married with more detailed epidemiological work and clinical studies, a series of hypotheses have been developed. At the broadest level such hypotheses suggest that 'multiple sclerosis [is] an acquired, exogenous [environmental] disease whose acquisition in ordinary circumstances takes place years before clinical onset' (Kurtzke 1980:78). This general hypothesis is reinforced by data which suggest that risk factors may be altered by migration at an appropriate age. Furthermore there is interesting evidence of 'epidemics' of multiple sclerosis. Kurtzke studied an epidemic of the disease in the Faroe Islands where a significant number of cases occurred (twenty-five) over the period 1943–70 following wartime British Army occupation (Kurtzke and Hyllested 1979). There was no evidence of the existence of multiple sclerosis before this period in the islands. It was thus hypothesized that the disease may be transmitted, which suggests a viral agent.

Much of the research on the causes of the disease has thus centred on strategies which seek either to identify directly a virus which might be implicated, or more indirectly define the precise circumstances in which such a virus (even if unidentified) might operate. Animal models have been widely employed in an attempt to understand the causative mechanisms and onset of diseases similar to multiple sclerosis, as well as to investigate the possibility that such diseases are transmittable to humans. In this respect a number of diseases of domestic and farm animals have received particular attention. For example there is active research still continuing on the association between specific diseases of sheep and multiple sclerosis, not least because of the remarkable correlation between the geographical distribution of sheep and the prevalence of multiple sclerosis (Murrell *et al.* 1986). However, the proof of a link remains at the level of epidemiological association, rather than of clear clinical evidence.

In the search for a viral explanation of the disease a 'sanitation hypothesis' about the cause of multiple sclerosis (Alter 1972) has been suggested. This was based on the substantial correlation between the prevalence of the disease and good sanitary conditions in many temperate countries. In such a situation many individuals might not be exposed to, and thus fail to gain immunity to, a putative multiple sclerosis virus in infancy. These individuals were thus likely to be particularly susceptible to later exposure to the slow-acting virus, perhaps between the ages of 5 and 15. However despite very considerable research effort, and the discovery of raised levels of antibodies in the blood of those with multiple sclerosis to, for example, measles virus, there has as yet been no clear evidence of a specific virus involved in the disease.

Another approach to identifying the cause of multiple sclerosis has been to concentrate on the immunological system, based on increasing evidence of some immunological breakdown in relation to the disease. This research does not preclude the possibility of a viral connection with multiple sclerosis, but seeks to study the pathological process of the disease from a complementary direction. It is not entirely clear whether the immunological problems occur before the onset of the disease, thus increasing susceptibility, or whether they are directly a consequence of the acquisition of multiple sclerosis. In either case research has been designed to discover the extent of immunological abnormality, and the mechanisms through which such abnormality occurs with the eventual hope of redressing the immunological balance in the body.

Following another line of enquiry, increasingly the causative relationship of nutrition to multiple sclerosis has come under scrutiny. High correlations have been demonstrated between the prevalence of the disease and the overall calorific intake, the intake of fats and oils, and the intake of calories of animal origin (Alter, Yamoor, and Harshe 1974: 268). Despite the relatively crude nature of the variables concerned, it has been hypothesized that a deficiency of certain dietary components, and an excess of others, may affect both the acquisition and the course of the disease. Interest has been particularly centred on the role of saturated animal fats on the one hand, and the role of essential fatty acids on the other hand. In those people with multiple sclerosis there are clear deficiencies of key fatty acids. Such deficiencies, if they occurred early in neural development, would in themselves present the possibility of abnormal nervous system growth and, if currently present, they would also make the likelihood of repair of damaged tissue – as in multiple sclerosis – less likely.

There have been many other theories about the cause of multiple sclerosis, based largely on epidemiological correlations, but also on particular sets of clinical observations. One theory is that multiple sclerosis has a vascular rather than a viral or immunological origin. Based on earlier speculations and on the similarity of many features of the pathology of multiple sclerosis to those of decompression sickness, James has argued that the disease may be caused by what he calls 'sub-acute fat embolism'

(1982: 380). In his view fat emboli cause damage to neurological tissue, in broadly the same way that gas embolism may do when diving with compressed air. Thus although the damage itself results in neurological symptoms, the fundamental cause of the damage is vascular. This view has not yet gained substantial currency amongst other medical researchers, although it is the subject of continuing interest (Poser 1986).

Aetiological theories have developed around such factors as the magnetic fields of the earth, microwave radiation, heavy metal pollution (leading to interest in mercury-based dental fillings) and many other possibilities. In the absence of decisive data a variety of theories will continue to be developed.

Finally it is important to note that despite the emphasis on exogenous factors as a cause of multiple sclerosis, there is an array of evidence that there is a genetic component in the aetiology of the disease. The strength of this genetic component is not entirely clear, or whether it operates completely independently of exogenous factors. An evaluation of the evidence up to 1982 by Spielman and Nathanson suggested that the frequency of the disease in siblings of those with multiple sclerosis is thirty times greater than for those in the general population, and fifteen times greater for parents and children (1982: 62). A simple genetic interpretation of this finding is not possible, and therefore much research has been undertaken on what genetic markers may be available to trace the disease.

It can be seen that the aetiology of multiple sclerosis continues to prove difficult to unravel. On the basis of the multiple lines of enquiry into the disease it appears that in all probability the cause will prove to be multi-factorial, involving both a genetic component, and what appears to be a more powerful array of exogenous or environmental factors. Further research is thus needed to elucidate the part that environmental as well as associated viral, immunological, nutritional, and biochemical factors play in the cause of the disease.

The medical management of multiple sclerosis

Given the unknown cause of the disease, as well as its relatively unpredictable course, the management of the condition is particularly problematic. Although in other conditions effective treatments have been discovered while the cause has still remained a mystery, in multiple sclerosis such a situation has not yet occurred. Consequently a wide array of potential treatments have been used; indeed Alter goes so far as to say that any treatment for any condition will sooner or later be applied to multiple sclerosis (1983).

There have been attempts to find treatments both for the disease itself, as well as effective means of managing the variety of symptoms which develop in its course. In the former area none has proved successful in the sense of providing the possibility of returning to the neurological state prior to the onset of the disease. This is in any event highly unlikely because of the intractability of neurological damage to repair. Thus most of the treatments have been designed to seek to prevent further development of the disease, while containing as far as possible the damage that has already been wrought.

One of the most widely used conventional therapies has been the administration of a corticosteroid (ACTH) which has been shown in clinical trials to reduce somewhat the length and severity of acute attacks in some patients. However it has not proved helpful for others, and has effects which make it unsuitable for long-term use. Another drug with broadly similar effects is prednisone, also used in acute attacks. Many of the drug therapies currently being assessed can be used only over limited periods of time, and their benefits generally appear to be temporary.

As a consequence of the difficulty of discovering effective long-term treatments for multiple sclerosis, much medical effort has been expended on finding means of relieving, as far as possible, some of the symptomatic consequences of the disease. General weakness, or tremor, as a result of multiple sclerosis has as yet little effective treatment, although there are encouraging results from the drug treatment of spasticity which often accompanies the disease. Other disturbances such as optic neuritis may be self-limiting in acute attacks, although often resulting in some residual impairment. There is little unequivocal evidence that optic neuritis can be aided by drug treatments; however some sensory problems may be alleviated to a degree, as may fatigue. A variety of ways of managing disturbances of the bowel and bladder are available either by the administration of drugs or by mechanical means. However, many of these managerial strategies are not entirely satisfactory – certainly from a patient's point of view – and may have to be adapted as dysfunctions increase and change with the development of the disease.

One of the consequences of the relatively limited armoury of conventional medical modes of managing multiple sclerosis has been the exploration of many alternative and unconventional therapies by people with the disease. These strategies may range from the adoption of sophisticated but medically unvalidated therapies, to a range of dietary and life-style changes. They are considered more fully in Chapter 5.

There is as yet no cure for multiple sclerosis. Treatments even in the broadest use of the word are relatively ineffective. The main emphasis of available therapies is therefore on the process of symptomatic relief. Even this limited objective can be only partially met at present.

The nature of multiple sclerosis

As was emphasized at the beginning of this chapter the phenomenon of multiple sclerosis presents major difficulties of interpretation, understanding, and management to both patients and doctors alike. Medical research and clinical work with the disease have led to gradually emerging knowledge, which currently is not sufficient to provide clear indications of effective treatment. Thus the combination of major medical problems associated with the disease, together with the relative paucity of the available therapies, tends to place patients and their families in a situation where they develop their own strategies for understanding and managing the consequences of the disease. It is the issues raised through this process that are now considered further.

Chapter two

Solving the puzzle: from the onset of symptoms to the diagnosis of multiple sclerosis

The symptomatic onset of multiple sclerosis can take many forms, both in the site and nature of individual symptoms, and in their mode of onset. The perception of these symptoms as medically significant, which warrant some explanation and action outside that normally given to the ordinary events of daily life, lies in the relationship between the nature of the symptoms and the individual's personal and social values and experiences. Mechanic (1978) has graphically indicated the wide range of non-medical factors which intercede in the definition of personal events and occurrences as symptoms of illness. These factors are associated, amongst other things, with the repetition, pain, unexpectedness, and suddenness of onset of the symptom, as well as the extent to which it interferes with the normal routines of life. Such factors are just as potent in the decision to seek the advice or help of others in relation to the recognized symptom. The threshold at which symptoms become perceptually visible is thus likely to vary considerably according to individual differences, and according to the social circumstances in which individuals are placed.

In the case of multiple sclerosis the variety of modes of onset of the disease is likely to enhance the probability that what later come to be recognized as serious symptoms are initially viewed as minor health problems resulting from the vagaries of life. Given the extent to which symptoms of all kinds are reported to be present in the general population the perception of the symptoms as of relatively little significance is not surprising. For example, 91 per cent of adults in Dunnell and Cartwright's survey reported an average of 3.9 symptoms each in the two weeks of the survey period; only 16 per cent had consulted a doctor (1972). Stewart and Sullivan (1982) indicate in their study how the insidious onset of symptoms of multiple sclerosis in many cases led to them initially being explained as 'non-serious' occurrences. They say:

> Instead of seeing their symptoms as indicative of serious illness, these patients viewed them as *ailments, minor illness or as symptoms of other treated illnesses, injuries or pregnancies.*
>
> (Stewart and Sullivan 1982: 1,399; emphasis in original)

With the widespread prevalence of minor symptoms similar to some of those experienced during the onset of multiple sclerosis, it is perhaps not surprising that those symptoms were interpreted in this way. Explanations in terms of overwork, tiredness, and being 'run down' were common in Stewart and Sullivan's study, as were accounts in terms of natural life stages such as, for example, 'getting older'. Several explanatory frameworks are readily available to individuals, subsequently diagnosed with multiple sclerosis, which draw on a common-sense range of assumptions about their initial symptoms. Such assumptions are far less likely to be used in relation to symptoms indicative of some other conditions where 'initial symptoms were severe, continuous, incapacitating and unalleviated' (Suchman 1965: 149).

In these circumstances rapid resort was made to medical advice. In contrast, the frequently variable and intermittent onset of multiple sclerosis allows the deployment of a far more eclectic set of interpretations.

For Susan the physical consequences of sport were sufficient to enable her to account for her first symptoms:

> We [Susan and her husband] had been to watch the film . . . and I could hardly walk into the bungalow in which we were staying. For the next two weeks my neighbour drove me to work because my legs remained stiff. I didn't tell my husband or the doctors at work because I assumed I had done too much tennis playing or swimming and had pulled the muscles.

Jane tried desperately to maintain the integrity of her body by characterizing her symptoms as mental aberrations:

> I think it started with me bumping into things with my left leg – then tripping up and falling over, and a peculiar sensation in the soles of my feet. . . . [However] I'd stand at the foot of the stairs and tell myself there's nothing wrong – it's all

in the mind, then up I'd go, and as was becoming usual practice
I'd trip and fall. . . . [I would say] I'm not doing it now –
there's nothing wrong – it will pass, but over I would go, again
and again – more bruises – and if anyone offered assistance
I would be angry and aggressive.

Sensory symptoms of an intermittent nature might be thought
easier to incorporate in everyday explanations than other events
of a dramatic kind – such as sudden loss or deterioration in sight
associated with optic neuritis. This latter occurrence appears to
herald the onset of the disease in perhaps 30 per cent of cases
(Matthews 1985: 97). Even in some of these situations where the
functional consequences of sudden visual loss would seem to be
severe, the context in which the symptom occurs may provide
a temporarily satisfactory interpretation of the event to those
concerned.

Catherine's comments indicate that loss of vision could be incorporated in her daily world. After several episodes when she
perceived her eyesight was deteriorating, she says:

Early in 1940 . . . I played in a netball match where as one
onlooker said 'You *were* that game'. My heart beat
excessively all that afternoon, but I cycled home and went out
in the evening. . . . I was a very active cyclist and went blind
pushing up a slope. I pulled to the gutter and waited for my
sight to return, which it did in a few minutes – perhaps my
ignorance was bliss then!

For many people apparently medically and functionally serious
symptoms at the onset of multiple sclerosis can be readily
explained or incorporated into everyday activities. They are
treated as an extension of the expected vagaries or excesses of
life. It appears to be their persistence over long periods of time,
their continual recurrence, an increase in their perceived seriousness, or the gradual appearance of other symptoms, which precipitate the quest for external help.

Seeking the help of others

The negotiation of the meaning of symptoms is also mediated
through the attitudes and beliefs of others. In particular where
symptoms are socially visible, either directly or through their func-

tional consequences, what has been described as the 'lay referral system' may be brought into play.

For John an observation by a colleague led him to reflect on his symptoms:

> Initially I had a strange ache constantly in my left forearm just below the elbow. I considered this to be merely a strain and then put it down to 'wear and tear'. After a few weeks the ache became more intense and seemed to occur above and below the elbow – although I couldn't establish exactly where. At the same time I began to have aches and pains around my neck and left shoulder. I put this down to sleeping posture and cramp.
>
> The symptoms referred to continued, sometimes more severe than others but always there. Then one day a lady colleague of mine suddenly said, 'Why are you walking with a limp?' 'Am I?' was the reply. It was after this that I realized that I was indeed walking with a slight limp on my left side. Within a week this became very noticeable. I found that I was unable to lift my left leg properly, and it was an effort climbing a flight of stairs.
>
> Strange as it now appears to me these various symptoms were very separate in my mind and no connection between them occurred to me at the time.

The advice of others, outside the medical system, may be sought deliberately after careful consideration. In the case of Geoff such advice was apparently in an unplanned way after a build-up of personal pressure:

> I returned to school and things really began to go wrong. A day at school would end and I would find myself collapsed in a chair, anxious and exhausted. I began to suffer from sudden 'jerks' in my arms and legs – later I was to discover these were spasms. Sometimes, my spine seemed to have a violently active life all its own; back-ache was almost constant; electric shocks seemed to run up my spine and into my skull. I suffered from extreme and vile headaches and nausea that left me totally exhausted. Things came to a head when one evening after school, in the presence of a teacher friend, I burst into tears. I explained that I didn't think I could go on any more, that everything was too much effort, and

that worst of all, I had no idea why. We discussed other aspects of my life which were settled and happy. I loved my job, my home, my friends and family. What was wrong?

Entering the medical system

In the case of those with early symptoms of multiple sclerosis, the usual mode of entry into the health-care system appears to be through a consultation with a general practitioner (Cunningham 1977; Stewart and Sullivan 1982). The circumstances in which this initial consultation occurs vary considerably. Often the consultation occurred as a result of an accretion of symptoms over a long period – in one study on average three years from their perceived beginning (Stewart and Sullivan 1982). The steady attrition of the plausibility of everyday explanations for the symptoms prompts a realization that the symptoms are not capable of acceptable interpretation in those ways, and may be serious. In addition the symptoms may begin to have such deleterious functional consequences at home or at work that medical advice is sought.

In contrast, where there are highly socially visible symptoms, particularly those which considerably disrupt trusted routines, entry into the health-care system is fast. Tom was underneath his car mending it when

> I just blacked out, my Dad dragged me . . . into my living room and lay me on my couch where if I moved my head half an inch I was violently sick . . . my GP was called out quickly.

However, the more usual pattern by which medical advice is sought is where it becomes increasingly difficult to continue to account plausibly for continuous but sporadic symptoms, as they materialize and intrude in daily living.

It would be a mistake however to conclude that the uncertainty and ambiguity which often characterizes the initial lay response to the early symptoms of multiple sclerosis is quickly resolved by contact with the medical system. Diffuse and intermittent symptoms, particularly those which can bear a variety of other medical interpretations, are not likely to be quickly or easily located by doctors as indicative of the disease. The classification and evaluation of such symptoms by general practitioners – the usual first point of medical contact – is a complex matter. Gale and Marsden (1985) point out several features of general practice which may lead to likely, perhaps even unavoidable, delays in definitive diagnosis. They note that contact with a wide range of problems, often of a general character, with limited access to immediate specialist knowledge, and with relatively little time for the detailed explorations of individual symptoms, may militate against an early clear diagnosis (1985: 64).

The evidence, in the cases of those subsequently diagnosed with multiple sclerosis, suggests that generally the first contact with the medical system does not lead quickly to a diagnosis, or even lead to a pathway through that system which could lead to a diagnosis. The first consultations can often appear to be satisfactory to both parties despite the failure to recognize the disease.

> The physicians either supported the patient's self-diagnoses or could find nothing physically wrong. At this point in the disease trajectory, such diagnoses were acceptable because patients also believed that nothing was seriously wrong. Normative consensus was easily accomplished because both patient and physician accepted the same definition of the patient's condition.
>
> (Stewart and Sullivan 1982: 1,400)

When an individual's medical history is complex there are often features that could legitimately be held to account for the appearance or exacerbation of symptoms, especially if they were of a kind related to temporary sensory loss. For Mary her problems began

> when I was suddenly unable to grip a pen, and workmates jokingly asked what I'd been drinking when my hand started shaking. At the same time I suffered severe pains in my head and neck, for which my GP prescribed pain-killers, which I took only when absolutely necessary. . . . At the same time I had trouble with my gums. The dentist assured me my teeth were perfect but I needed an operation called Gingevectomy. This operation was carried out under local anaesthetic at a Dental Hospital, and I confess I went through hell. . . . All in all 1975 was a dreadful year. Could my aches, pains, and tremors just be a nervous reaction from the mouth operations which were quite traumatic? . . . By 1976 my mouth had

healed . . . and the doctor assured me that the pains in my
neck and lack of grip were just a touch of arthritis, and I
should keep taking the pain-killers.

This account both demonstrates the plausibility of alternative
explanations for early symptoms of multiple sclerosis and also the
gradual realization on the patient's part that those explanations
were becoming less credible. Other accounts stress the way that
explanatory consensus between doctor and patient is reached by
reference to the anticipated and 'ordinary' effects of particular life
stages, life events, or various precipitating factors.

Some symptoms may be directly perceived as indicating the
presence of depressive or other mental illness and be treated
accordingly. Thus Chris notes:

I became ill in 1975–6 with difficult-to-identify symptoms,
some of which seem now clearly to be MS. At the time I was
working in the evening, as well as the day, and doing up a
house as well. . . . I saw a doctor and was treated for
depression, after which I did become depressed. In a way I
felt this was partly because I had lost credence – people
didn't believe in me anymore so I took the opportunity to let
go of the reins and let others take over. Anyway I felt and
I still do that I was able to sustain the pace and that wasn't
just why I was so weak and 'ill feeling'. . . . However I took
the treatment and the label.

The failure to recognize the symptoms in these accounts as indicative of multiple sclerosis by both physicians and patients is not
surprising.

First, all the accounts are retrospective. The reconstruction of
personal biographies following a diagnosis of the disease involves,
amongst other things, a review and re-evaluation of symptoms
previously regarded as minor, and arising from other causes.

Second, as has been indicated before, the multiplicity and
nature of the symptoms which may be registered by people at the
onset of the disease could be legitimately liable to a wide range
of medical interpretations. Statistically more common explanations may therefore be initially employed in these circumstances, rather than that of multiple sclerosis. In addition, as
diagnostic criteria for multiple sclerosis stress the need to register

the existence of discrete episodes of the illness over time, multiple medical assessments before diagnosis are likely.

Third, as Gale and Marsden (1985) suggest, immediate management of the symptoms may be the general practitioners' major concern. Symptoms, other than of an acute and serious kind, may be treated at first as discrete and liable either to spontaneous remission – a particular characteristic of many symptoms of the disease – or as amenable to minor medical palliatives.

Fourth, it is important to realize that there may be other diseases, conditions, or states existing concurrently with the development of multiple sclerosis. Discrimination between such states and the symptoms of multiple sclerosis may require a finesse of judgement and knowledge not available, or called upon, in the early stages of the disease.

The medical merry-go-round

An initial mis-diagnosis, or non-diagnosis of multiple sclerosis, at the point of first medical contact may be explained by reference to some of the factors enumerated above. The processes operating from that point initiate a new phase in the relationship between physicians and patients. From a broadly consensual relationship there may develop one of doubt, mistrust, and conflict as patients become dissatisfied with physicians' understanding of their condition. Stewart and Sullivan argue that there is an increasing discrepancy between the patient's perception of the severity and functional impact of his or her symptoms, and the plausibility of the medical explanations received for them (1982: 1,400). The patient's quest is therefore to find medical explanations of the situation which are congruent with his or her own view of its seriousness and origins. This quest is described by Cunningham as resulting in 'a medical merry-go-round' (1977: 24).

There are a number of related aspects to this process which it is important to consider. First, there may be clinical uncertainty as to a definitive diagnosis resulting in physician-initiated referrals through the medical system. That uncertainty may be prolonged in many cases either because of the need to ascertain two or more episodes of the disease, or through an inability to make an early differential diagnosis. Second, there may be a definite clinical diagnosis made of multiple sclerosis which is not communicated to the patient, or a diagnosis made of some other condition, both situations being deemed unsatisfactory by the patient, resulting in patient-prompted referrals through the medical system.

From a patient's perspective, in the short term it may be difficult or perhaps practically impossible to determine which situation he or she is in. In an attempt to resolve this position Stewart and Sullivan argue that patients subsequently diagnosed as having multiple sclerosis increasingly take an active and less deferential role in the medical system (1982: 1,401). The paradox is, however, that uncertainty for most can only be resolved through a further medical encounter. Finding the 'right' doctor to provide this resolution satisfactorily can be a lengthy task. Whether the 'merry-go-round' is physician initiated through clinical uncertainty, or patient prompted through what F. Davis (1960) calls functional uncertainty or a perceived mis-diagnosis, the number and variety of medical contacts in the early stages of multiple sclerosis is likely to be considerable.

Ruth went through a set of hospital consultations and tests initiated by her general practitioner when she contacted him again after 'putting her feet up' didn't work:

> By August I was afraid to walk down a slope, and found an incline or stairs difficult. So once again I went to see my GP who arranged an appointment at the neurology department at my local hospital.
>
> Early September found me at the hospital for my initial test, and after answering a few questions and walking a few steps, I was staggered to be asked to arrange for a week's stay in hospital for further tests. So a week later I was back again. . . . Then followed lumbar puncture, brain scan, myelogram, blood tests, etc. I was dismayed to learn of the many nervous diseases and their various effects. . . . It is enough to say I didn't enjoy my stay in hospital, but I was sent home with the knowledge that I had an infection in my spine. After hospital followed a daily injection at home of ACTH. . . . There followed two weeks without injections, and a further report back to hospital. When I saw the specialist he thought I was much better . . . and could return to the office. This I did working few hours, but found this even together with the travelling too much, so I once again sought medical help.

At the end of this process she had been told 'a holding diagnosis', but did not appear nearer to receiving the formal diagnosis of multiple sclerosis.

Alistair adopted a forthright strategy in his approach to his doctor, but eventually turned to alternative approaches outside conventional medicine:

> My left foot started to drag and I had difficulty in walking. I could not raise my right arm . . . and I could not make the fourth and fifth fingers in my left hand strike the keys on my typewriter.
>
> During the next six months my left arm and leg became more and more useless but the doctor said it was strained muscles. At the end of six months I said I must see a specialist and was sent to a neurologist in the local town. I was taken to a nursing home for tests but nothing definite emerged. Nothing definite did later, although I went for tests a year later at another hospital. Both these spells in hospital made me feel a lot worse and since then I have steered clear of them. I have now on the other hand tried acupuncture, the Alexander treatment, relaxation, faith-healing, and massage. None of these things made me feel any better, although I think that talking to people did me more good than anything else.

The gradual realization of the increasing discrepancy between their own perception of the disintegrating integrity of their bodily processes, and medical explanations of them, has, in these cases, led to a variety of strategies to overcome this dissonance. The main strategy, despite the concern with the validity of individual medical judgements, is to seek a satisfactory endorsement using the powerful legitimizing role of the medical profession. This not only ensures a greater congruence between patients' perceptions and a professional judgement, but also allows the assumption of an acceptable sick role amongst family, friends, and relatives (Stewart and Sullivan 1982: 1,401). The negotiation of such a role may be vital in the re-establishment of a tolerable personal and social life, whether or not individual symptoms and their consequences can be effectively treated.

The medical merry-go-round is thus likely to be a continuing feature of the quest for a diagnosis of multiple sclerosis. It may be propelled either by a medical concern to reduce clinical uncertainty, or the concern, by the patient, to eliminate diagnoses they deem not commensurate with their symptoms, or to make explicit diagnoses they believe have been made but not disclosed.

The discovery of the diagnosis of multiple sclerosis

The discovery of the diagnosis of multiple sclerosis is a point of major significance in the personal biography of those with the disease, and their families. Such a discovery may be an event simultaneous with the formal medical confirmation, but the discovery may precede the latter. One study suggests that approximately a third of those with multiple sclerosis had discovered the diagnosis before being told by their medical adviser (I. Robinson 1983). Three further studies indicate that the revelation of the diagnosis of multiple sclerosis by doctors is often undertaken belatedly, and in ways in which uncertainty about the nature of the disease is maximized for patients (Scheinberg *et al.* 1984; Elian and Dean 1985; Radford and Trew 1987). Scheinberg and his colleagues express their concern that the previous efforts of patients attending their medical centre to find the meaning of their symptoms often yielded 'unsatisfactory outcomes' such as the use of inaccurate or euphemistic names for the disease; the generation of fears in patients that doctors were unable or unwilling to make a diagnosis; or the use of unnecessary and sometimes hazardous diagnostic tests (1984: 205).

In the light of the discussion in this chapter these outcomes should occasion little surprise – reflecting the consequences of both clinical and managerial uncertainty. However a series of significant issues are raised by the delays and difficulties experienced around the revelation of the diagnosis.

Elian and Dean (1985) document the extent to which individual entrepreneurship, as well as chance encounters, had been used by patients in the pursuit of their diagnosis. Overheard conversations, overseen medical notes, and apparently accidental revelations in conversations with paramedical staff and others had all resulted in discoveries of the diagnosis. Such discoveries had been accomplished outside the medically anticipated framework of a formal revelation and discussion by a consultant neurologist. An editorial in the *Lancet* commenting on the findings of Elian and Dean suggested that

It is indefensible on ethical or humanitarian grounds that

patients should be left to make one of the most devastating discoveries of their lives by accident without any professional support or evaluation.

The editorial emphasized the importance of an early indication of the diagnosis to the patient, but was careful to circumscribe this both with the need to ensure clinical certainty about the diagnosis, and with the need to endorse the freedom of clinical judgement in the matter.

It does appear that many, perhaps the vast majority of, physicians say they always or often tell the patient their diagnosis of multiple sclerosis (in Scheinberg *et al.*'s study it was 97 per cent – 1984: 209). This may represent a major change in previous attitudes towards disclosure, if the changes in physicians' attitudes towards the disclosure of diagnoses of cancer are replicated (Oken 1961; Novack *et al.* 1979). However, the statements of physicians about their practices, and the reports from patients about their knowledge of their diagnoses, suggest a discrepancy between physician-expressed intention and physician behaviour. Scheinberg *et al.* indicate that this discrepancy may arise through physicians' delaying disclosure on the basis of their judgement of the patient's intelligence; age; emotional stability; degree of emotional support; medical sophistication; and the wishes of the relatives (1984: 209). Such a considerable array of factors could delay the revelation of the diagnosis in many, perhaps most, cases.

In addition following the problems that may stem from clinical uncertainty, the disclosure of a diagnosis may be delayed through a physician's judgement of how a patient may react to that disclosure. Further it may well be that other considerations reinforce a tendency to delay disclosure. Glaser indicates how the potential emotional resource and practical costs of the disclosure for the physician may delay disclosure of a diagnosis (1972: 194). This factor, in addition to those above, could contribute to the problems found to be associated with the diagnosis of multiple sclerosis.

The absence of any clear path of treatment or management following the formal diagnosis of multiple sclerosis may also inhibit its early revelation to the patient. At one extreme some diagnoses will confer

a sound prediction of the course the disease will take, will imply its etiology, and perhaps most important of all it will suggest the course of treatment that will later alter its progression. The value of making such a diagnosis increases with the definiteness with which such predictions are possible once the diagnosis is made.

(Mechanic 1978: 96)

The diagnosis of multiple sclerosis implies little knowledge about any of the components mentioned by Mechanic, and is associated consequently with few standard and medically positive courses of action. Thus the 'instrumental' reasons perceived by doctors for the early revelation of the diagnosis are relatively few in the case of multiple sclerosis.

With the common lengthy history of symptoms, and attempts at their explanation by the patient and their family, it is not surprising that patients may alight, in the end, on multiple sclerosis as a possible interpretation of the phenomena which beset them independently of their medical advisers. There are a variety of ways in which the discovery of the diagnosis may be achieved (Elian and Dean 1985; I. Robinson 1983; Radford and Trew 1987). Parallels may be drawn between the symptoms of friends or acquaintances with multiple sclerosis and their own situation, or from textbook descriptions, or from interviews, conversations, or reports on radio, television, or in the newspapers.

For example George said:

I guessed after reading the article in the *Readers Digest*. I mentioned this to my sister and then she told me that my guess was correct as my father had told her.

June indicated that she

had a slight suspicion that I might have MS after reading an article in a magazine about a model who had MS. I did not have all the symptoms she had, but I had enough to make me wonder. In fact the next time I had to see the consultant I almost asked him if I had got MS but decided not to as I'd had lots of tests whilst in hospital and he would have known if I had MS and would have told me. At that stage I had no idea that the doctor would not tell me as soon as he knew.

Scheinberg *et al.* (1984) note that in 25 per cent of cases in their study the neurologist informed relatives first of the diagnosis – sometimes with the instruction that the patients should not themselves be told. In some cases there was an attempt to 'manage the discovery' of the diagnosis so that the formal disclosure should be a relatively painless affair, a matter of routine confirmation. This appears to be more common in cases where women are diagnosed with multiple sclerosis.

Peggy illustrates how this process works:

At the first consultation with the neurologist at the age of 19 years my mother asked him point blank if the diagnosis was multiple sclerosis. He evaded a direct reply launching into an explanation of multiple sclerosis. He said he preferred to call my condition a virus infection of the central nervous system, and that with the treatment he was going to prescribe, namely ACTH, there was a 98 per cent chance of recovery. I left the consulting room somewhat confused, as indeed my parents were when we discussed it six months later. . . . During these months after treatment and because the symptoms continued I concluded myself that multiple sclerosis was the only possible diagnosis. Although the specialist had avoided giving me the true diagnosis he made himself available for consultation whenever I asked, to discuss my condition. I had the impression that he wanted me to work it out for myself – probably his way of lessening the blow.

This strategy may also fail when the person subject to the diagnosis strongly resents what may be seen as a patronizing attitude to them and their life by doctors and/or their relatives. In some cases the diagnosis contained in medical records may be divulged in unforeseen circumstances by other medical or paramedical staff who have access to those records, for example by physiotherapists, occupational therapists, or nurses (Elian and Dean 1985). In other cases the trust between doctor and patient or between husband and wife may be shattered. Rosalyn describes her continuing resentment that her husband was told before she was:

I was staggered when I found that he [her husband] had been told before me. Moreover he had known for six months and had been told not to tell me. I do not feel I can trust either my doctor or him any more – it has completely changed our relationship.

Reconstructing biographies: from symptoms to diagnosis

In this chapter the trajectory of those subsequently diagnosed as having multiple sclerosis has been described from the onset of their symptoms to the diagnosis itself. This trajectory, conditioned as it is by the variable and intermittent character of the disease, as well as the many social and personal settings in which it occurs, is a multifaceted one. In this process many everyday 'common-sense' explanations may be used which appear to account for the initial symptoms, however they are subsequently discarded. The introduction of family, friends, and medical advice into this interpretative process, which can often initially bear equally plausible interpretations, may not lead to an early satisfactory explanation of the pattern of events associated with the symptoms.

Many of those subsequently diagnosed as having multiple sclerosis have medical histories of great complexity in which the diagnosis of the disease emerges in a variety of ways. The circumstances in which the diagnosis is discovered or disclosed appear to be of considerable importance in influencing the strategies through which the disease and its consequences are managed by patients and their families. These issues are considered in the next chapter.

Chapter three

Life with multiple sclerosis: subjective experience and the disease

Being a person with multiple sclerosis: personal reactions to the disease

The experience of the discovery of the diagnosis is as crucial to the patient with the disease as is the making of the diagnosis for the physician. For the physician the diagnosis represents in summary form a complex pattern of medical judgements about signs and symptoms (Mishler 1981: 144–9).

For the patient, the diagnosis formally incorporates their symptoms within a legitimizing framework, externally validating their status as a 'sick person'. The conferring of the diagnosis on a person with multiple sclerosis has been viewed as the end to a lengthy period of fraught negotiation (Stewart and Sullivan 1982: 1,402).

Research on patients' experience of the revelation of a diagnosis suggests that a number of consequences are particularly important. Many of these stem from the social and personal effects of medical legitimizing. The formal medical classification of an array of symptoms can provide a socially acceptable means of incorporating those symptoms into everyday life. The 'label' of the diagnosis is thus a basis on which to develop more visible managerial strategies – particularly in the diagnosis of a condition with little stigma attached to it. However the 'label' may, at the same time, constrain and restrict those possibilities where the diagnosis is of a more stigmatized condition. Comparing the revelation of the diagnosis in the case of multiple sclerosis with that in the case of epilepsy some important differences emerge. In Scambler's study reactions to the diagnosis of epilepsy were shock and concern; 'almost without exception, people were extremely upset when the diagnostic label was applied' (1984: 212). People were shocked because they felt that the diagnosis had 'in an important way, made them into epileptics . . . [a] stigmatising condition' (Scambler 1984: 213).

In the case of multiple sclerosis the reactions of those to whom the diagnosis has been revealed can be profoundly different. The lengthy and complicated initial course of many people with the disease has already been discussed, and this trajectory appears to be associated with a more complex response to the diagnosis than is shown in Scambler's study.

An indication of an unexpectedly positive response to the revelation of the medically serious diagnosis of multiple sclerosis is given in the study by Cunningham (1977). She indicates that ten out of the sixteen cases she interviewed 'claimed to have experienced relief once they were given the diagnosis' (1977: 30). Cunningham is unsure whether these accounts of relief are

> part of the strategies used by multiple sclerosis patients in an attempt to deny the real significance of the disease . . . [but it was clear that] the disclosure of the diagnosis gave back to many of the respondents their credibility and legitimised their strange behaviours which had previously been labelled as neurotic, hypochondria, malingering or drunk.
>
> (Cunningham 1977: 31)

Another study based on a far larger population also found that feelings of relief were indicated by a majority (53 per cent) of those receiving the diagnosis (I. Robinson 1983: 19). Such feelings may be explained in either of the ways that Cunningham describes, but the discovery, after a lengthy period of concern, of a less stigmatized condition, or a less immediately serious diagnosis than that feared – such as a brain tumour – may be particularly likely to occasion the sense of relief.

These findings must not, however, be taken as indicating that the diagnosis of multiple sclerosis is universally and unequivocally greeted with a sense of relief. Grief, anger, fear, and shock are all experienced, in varying proportions, by those given the diagnosis of multiple sclerosis (I. Robinson 1983: 19). But the giving of the diagnosis cannot be assumed to be an entirely negative event for all those to whom it is revealed, or to be completely 'bad news', as a number of the accounts below indicate.

A very positive view of the giving of the diagnosis is given by Margaret, who writes:

'You have multiple sclerosis,' the doctor at the hospital said – I couldn't wait to get out of the out-patients' department. Once in the car I turned to my husband and said gleefully, 'Thank God, I now know what's wrong with me, I'm so pleased.' You see I had been under the hospital for two years, had test after test, and been in and out a couple or so times and on my two monthly appointments had always asked, 'What's wrong with me?', only to be told, 'We are not sure. We have to be certain'. So I asked to be told what I hadn't got – to no avail. Now I knew and I could tell people who asked what was wrong with me – I was not imagining things, or going mental – Yippee!

May experienced both shock and relief at the point of the discovery of her diagnosis:

It was at the third follow-up visit that I asked the neurologist directly if I had MS. He said, 'Yes'. Although I had felt more or less convinced for some time that this was so, it still came as a bit of a shock to be told officially. Yet in some ways it was also a relief; it provided what seemed to me a logical reason for all my peculiar symptoms and the everlasting tiredness.

For others shock was the dominant emotion experienced at the time of the revelation of the diagnosis. This shock appears to be occasioned either by a very rapid transition from a relatively symptom-free state to being given the diagnosis, or a well-developed and frightening image of what someone with the disease would be like. In either situation the implied consequences for social and personal life are perceived as very substantial, and almost entirely negative. Terry's wife describes how they reacted to the discovery of his diagnosis:

The news came so unexpectedly and shocked us so much that for a long time we were unable to think clearly. . . . He [Terry] only knew that MS is considered the second most feared disease! . . . for several months he and I suffered terribly.

In the case of Claire the shock appeared to be occasioned particu-

larly by the relatively quick transition from a symptomless state
to the discovery of the diagnosis. After an intensive series of tests
in hospital after her first symptoms, and a course of ACTH, Claire
was told by a registrar she

> had an incurable disease, which they didn't know the name
> of, but I had one consolation, it wouldn't kill me! I decided
> to see another neurologist. My GP gave me a letter to take
> to him; when I got it home I steamed it open to discover I
> had MS. What a shock, it was awful . . . it took me a long
> time before I did anything about it [her MS].

Overall, first reactions to the diagnosis of multiple sclerosis are
conditioned by many factors. One of the most important is the
patient's trajectory before the point at which the diagnosis is
revealed. In one study 57 per cent of those diagnosed with multiple
sclerosis considered they did not discover that diagnosis until five
years or more had elapsed from their first suspected symptom,
while over a third had discovered their diagnosis before being
formally told (I. Robinson 1983: 7–9). It is thus not surprising
that at the time they were formally told, reactions to the diagnosis
of a serious medical condition would not necessarily be those that
were expected by physicians.

Mobilizing personal resources: managing the experience of multiple sclerosis

How people with multiple sclerosis redesign their lives, given the
diagnosis, is a matter of debate. No unequivocally agreed and
common explanatory framework has been devised. However,
managing 'the crisis of chronic illness' – frequently a situation of
serious personal disequilibrium – has been discussed using the
idea of coping mechanisms (DiMatteo and Friedman 1982: 181–2).
The importance of this approach is that it is based on the view
that it is the *personal interpretation* of events, rather than the
events themselves, which is significant.

Individual strategies, in this view, are seen to depend on
people's personal reaction to the presence of the disease. Matson
and Brooks, for example, suggest four different reactions may
occur in response to multiple sclerosis, which they indicate are
likely to be experienced sequentially. They consider that people
may first deny the disease – 'It's not true'; then they may resist

the disease – 'I will fight it'; then they may affirm the disease – 'I have to accept it'; then they may integrate the disease into their lives – 'It's there but only part of my life' (1977: 249). Each of these reactions in their turn are associated with major differences in life strategy.

Matson and Brooks imply that the four-stage model is useful as a guide to a putative transition from denial (stage 1), through stages 2 and 3 to stage 4 (integration). They seem to feel that this sort of transition would be a sign of positive and successful adjustment to the disease. However, in their two studies there is little evidence of such a transition being a common pattern; nor of those following that pattern being more 'successfully' adjusted than those who do not; nor of any clear link between degree of physical disability, length of time with the disease, and the stage reached in the model (1977: 250). The problem of setting up such a model is that others, such as Vanderplate (1984: 265), have given it a status and a definitive role in understanding reactions to the disease, which no empirical research has yet substantiated. It seems therefore that the idea that length of time with the disease or degree of disability in themselves condition reactions, or life strategies, must be treated with some scepticism. Matson and Brooks argue that other factors, such as psycho-social ones, must be considered, particularly those which relate to personal attitudes and those which relate to the social context in which multiple sclerosis is perceived. Even so these psycho-social factors appear to operate in ways which preclude an easy explanation of the personal process undergone by people with the disease.

The question of how people with multiple sclerosis personally deal with the challenge posed by the disease is taken up in a more pragmatic way in the work of Pollock (1984). Of the four categories mentioned by Matson and Brooks she pays particular attention to the ways in which people resist or fight the disease, although without considering this issue as part of a sequence of events. Indeed, in comparing people with schizophrenia, with the onset of a neurotic disorder (described as nervous breakdown), and with multiple sclerosis, she concludes that it was characteristic of those with multiple sclerosis that they believed that attitude of mind could be effectively applied against the disease.

In Pollock's study resistance was the major strategy pursued by those with multiple sclerosis, despite the belief by others that many had 'given in'. The strategies of denial, acceptance, or integration were less frequently and less readily adopted.

In another study, the strategy of 'fighting' the disease was most often perceived in the response of people with multiple sclerosis to their situation. Over half of the spouses in this study felt that their partners with the disease were 'fighting' it, as opposed to any other strategy (Robinson 1988). This approach to resisting multiple sclerosis indicates that a special relationship is assumed to exist between body and mind in containing, controlling, or 'beating' the disease. Such a strategy operates not only through emphasizing the active role of individuals in their choice of therapeutic regime, but also through the perceived benefits of this vigorous and unyielding state of mind itself.

The views of Robin illustrate the kinds of processes that may prompt this strategy. He felt himself faced with stark options. For example Robin states his choices as

(1) Accept the disease (2) Kill myself or (3) Fight it. I considered all three seriously. I thought through what was going to happen with the MS. In the end I decided that I wasn't going to accept it – I'd always been a battler and I could never just sit back and let it happen. The thought of killing myself was a real possibility; I couldn't bear to be crippled when I'd been so active, and my wife wouldn't have to look after me. But I felt that, in the end, that was also giving in to MS. I then determined that I was going to fight it every day, and find everything and anything that could put it in its place. It was not going to win.

Stan considered two choices, but really had no doubts about which one he would choose, based on his explanation of multiple sclerosis. His battle was not with some abstract, fortuitous, and inexorable disease process, but with a personalized intruder – indeed an intruder which he himself had invited, or had left the door open for. His choice was

To accept it or to fight it. . . . [I will not accept it because] I am too busy living to wait [for a cure]. I have never been healthier in body and mind. *I believe the cure lies in the power of the individual.* I got myself sick, I'll get myself better. The fact that no research has really been able to prove anything is proof in itself that the cure is not going to come through a miracle drug for everyone, because everyone does not have the same symptoms. What has worked for some in putting MS into remission has not worked for others. It appears to me the disease is too specific – too suited to the individual. It requires a one-to-one approach. I have heard similar thoughts expressed in the saying 'Never give up, you can beat it'.

Denial, acceptance, and integration, the remaining three of the Matson and Brooks categories, appear to be less frequently employed. However three points must be recognized here.

First, the social visibility of those who are 'fighting' the disease may be greater than those following other strategies. This resistance itself may lead to demonstrable – sometimes dramatic – lifestyle changes and an active, involved, and continuous search for therapies to manage the disease. Such an approach – discussed more fully in Chapter 5 – is more likely to be amenable to research, than those strategies which are based on or are associated with more discreet and less publicly identifiable behaviour.

Second, what precisely constitutes 'denial', as opposed to 'acceptance' for example, is at the margin a matter of considerable debate. In Matson and Brooks's terms denial relates to a refusal to believe that the disease is present at all. However, the disease may be accepted as being present and the diagnosis as being 'true', while its specific physical effects may be denied. Or even if those specific physical effects are accepted, their functional impact may be denied. Or even if the functional impact is accepted, their personal and social relevance may be denied. Thus denial may occur in different ways, in which an analytical – and empirical – separation from other strategies is difficult to achieve.

Third, and perhaps most important, it may be fallacious to conceive of a single dominant strategy being employed at all – despite the observations above. 'Fighting' or 'resisting' the disease may itself co-exist side by side with elements of denial, acceptance, or integration. Those who fight the disease in one context may deny it in another and accept it in yet another.

An indication of how elements of denial, acceptance, and resistance may be incorporated in a personal strategy is provided by Dana who, whatever the external judgements may be, appears to consider herself as having integrated the disease into her life:

I think I have accepted it [multiple sclerosis] very well. I have become a very determined person and a strong positive thinker. I do not allow anything to get me down now, and I am determined never to let myself go. I have also started to go out and meet new people and begin my life again. I am determined that no one will think there is anything wrong with me. I have also decided to spend a lot of time in finding out what I could do for myself. I was not going to sit at home and wait for something to happen. I also realized that I was on my own with this problem, but I am going to fight it even on my own now.

No doubt such an account could be characterized as belonging more to one of the strategies which has been discussed than another. However it is crucial that such a characterization does not understate the complexity of the strategies which individuals may deploy, nor their dynamic character. Such strategies may only occasionally unfold in the discrete, uniform, and linear way suggested by the coping model of Matson and Brooks.

Uncertainty: managing the past, present, and future

The uncertainty which attends the early history of many patients with multiple sclerosis has been argued by Stewart and Sullivan to be largely resolved by the discovery of the diagnosis (1982: 1,402–3). However uncertainty and ambiguity in other forms are not resolved so easily. As Blaxter points out prognostic uncertainty is not necessarily resolved by the diagnosis (1976: 233). In the case of multiple sclerosis there is no definitive and clear prognosis that can be given for any particular patient, except in general that the disease is likely to be progressive at some unspecified rate. There is thus considerable latitude for the interpretation of the future course of the disease by both patient and physician.

In this setting uncertainty as to the present or future course of the disease – and its effects on anticipated, expected, or desired personal or social goals – has to be managed. Wright notes that in entering the new situations continually created in this process, each attempt to move towards a desired goal may have both positive and negative effects (1983: 109).

In conditions of uncertainty, with a disease like multiple sclerosis, it may be difficult to evaluate what is the most appropriate course of action to achieve a goal – especially so where the anticipated costs of failure are high. Wright considers that there are three major types of ambiguities in any new situation. Each requires interpretation as to their costs and benefits. The first of these is the uncertainty of whether a situation can be physically managed; the second is uncertainty over the reaction of others; the third is uncertainty about the self-concept of the person concerned (1983: 109).

Hirsch describes the physical parameters of this uncertainty in a vivid fashion:

> With a progressive disease like multiple sclerosis . . . it's necessary that year after year, month after month, sometimes week after week, new adaptations have to be made, adaptations which can last only as long as the condition remains the same. Since, even with a plateau, the condition does not remain the same for very long, new adaptations constantly have to be instituted. Perhaps worst of all it is not knowing how things will eventually end. Will I be totally helpless? Will I be bedridden? Will I be able to move at all? By constant adaptation I mean that as one problem is vanquished and as peace is made with regard to it, this problem gives way to a new one, and this problem in its turn gives way to another one, only for another to take its place. Thus walking normally gives way to walking with a cane, the cane gives way to a walker, the walker gives way to pushing oneself in a wheelchair, and pushing oneself finally gives way to being pushed by another person. Similarly writing gives way to typing, which gives way to printing, which gives way to only scrawling one's signature.
>
> (Hirsch 1977: 151–2, quoted in Wright 1983: 111)

Anticipating the likely chain of physical events may be a means of attempting to reduce the range of uncertainty in this developing situation. However, such a strategy does not have a great chance of success. Strauss points out that what they describe as 'imaginary rehearsals of future events' involves an interplay between the course of the illness as it unfolds, and the personal trajectory of the individual person concerned – that is the life consequences and meaning attributed to that illness. It may be, they argue, that the course of the illness is so rapid and unexpected that it overtakes people's anticipatory work, or on the other hand that the anticipation is, in effect, redundant (1984: 65–7). When considering multiple sclerosis either, or indeed both, possibilities may prove to be the case at different points in a life with the disease. Thus uncertainty about the future physical depredations of this condition may be sustained. The apparently steady physical progression that Hirsch notes above is not typical of all cases of the disease (Kraft *et al.* 1981), and his description may more closely reflect his own personal trajectory than the general course of multiple sclerosis.

Continuing uncertainty about the reaction of others, the second of Wright's categories, remains problematic for many. The multiplicity of symptoms that may characterize the disease, their variability, and particularly their differing social visibility, can lead to substantial discrepancies between self-perceptions and the perception of others. Even when the diagnosis is known, symptoms which may not always be socially obvious – such as incontinence or fatigue – or symptoms which appear and disappear in the early stages of the disease may make it difficult to be accepted as 'really sick' in everyday life. Thus despite having a medical imprimatur confirming the diagnosis, the powerful but often understated scepticism of others perpetuates the uncertainties felt by those with multiple sclerosis about the nature of their situation. Blaxter found that a number of people with early multiple sclerosis felt that they might be stigmatized because their symptoms made them 'strange and difficult to understand' (1976: 202).

Rosie writes that

> most non-MS people know very little about the disease, unless they have been close to someone who has it, and, in my particular situation, . . . I *look* fairly fit and healthy, and no one can *see* the ache in my legs, the 'funny sensations' and the tiredness.

In the case of Sarah her incontinence was her most problematic symptom and had led her to be socially isolated because she felt that

> No one else can really understand unseen symptoms like tiredness and incontinence. My husband, and our friends, can't understand why I don't want to go out as often as they would like. They feel that I should make the effort, but I would have to go out with a bag full of pads and pants in case

I can't get to a toilet in time. I can't really explain what it is like.

Indeed one of the problems appears to be that so many of the symptoms of the disease, at least in the early stages, are in effect 'exaggerated' versions of conditions experienced by many people in the rough and tumble of everyday life. Therefore the discrepancy between personal and social perceptions, and the uncertainty generated through this discrepancy, may be sustained long after the diagnosis is revealed.

The third of Wright's categories, that is the uncertainty about self-image, is one which may be a constant problem with multiple sclerosis. Strauss locates the issue of the uncertainty of self-image firmly in the context of what they call 'social arrangements' and social relationships (1984: 73). For them self-image is a product of the reciprocal but changing association between people with chronic disease and those around them. The question of 'Who am I?' is thus produced out of a dialogue with who other people think you are. Living with multiple sclerosis generates a constant re-evaluation of that question. Gemma, reflecting on her relationships with her family, feels she has positively integrated uncertainty into those relationships:

> I find it difficult to say exactly how things are. I have been through so many phases of the illness, where both my feelings and their reactions change sometimes for the better, and sometimes for the worse. At first it was very hard, as I began to decline, their attitude was one of complete indifference whilst they still expected me to do the same. . . . I knew I wasn't the same as I used to be . . . but they didn't want their lives altered in any way even though they knew I had MS. As they did more I did less. MS does alter your life and that of those around you and you all have to accept this. As things change they have become more aware of me and my feelings, and about what I can and can't do. I feel it's much easier now.

Chris feels, conversely, that the continuing uncertainty has constantly undermined her efforts to sustain her self-image:

> [Looking back] I don't remember much about the MS episodes, as they all blur into the crowding of the recent years. I've been moved in my job several times, which is

because of the MS, as my employers feel that I must be put in a job where it won't matter too much if I should be ill. In a way that's made me lose self-respect. . . . I'm afraid to presume on it [life] as I have before and things have fallen apart. . . . I would not know how to say that I have come to terms with what has happened to me. I don't know that I have ever come to terms with things, they push me down for a while whilst I try to work out what is happening, then I surface again until the next lot happens . . . there seem to be so many things going on that I feel bamboozled.

Many of the issues thrown up by these uncertainties relate to what has been called 'the delicately balanced game of temporal juggling' (Strauss 1984: 62). In the case of multiple sclerosis the juggling lies in the management of relationships between the past, the present, and the future – between what was, what is, and what could be. Where future uncertainty is magnified, the present, reinterpreted through the past, is a more attractive – perhaps the only attractive – proposition. Adrienne indicates how she feels:

it is true to say that this illness has permeated my life and had a profound effect on me even though I am not physically disabled. It has altered my perception of my future and has forced me to be less ambitious particularly in career terms. The changes are not all negative ones. I now have a heightened sense of living in and enjoying the present. My motivation to get and stay fit has never been higher and I am reaping the benefits of a healthy life-style. I try hard not to use MS as an excuse to opt out of living (as I have seen some people no worse than me doing) but at the same time I try to be sensible and realistic about my activities and aims in life. No one knows what the future holds for them. I am relying on continuing to be one of the lucky ones.

Such a view, expressing a common theme in autobiographical accounts, is articulated more briefly by Pam:

I don't really want to think too much about the future. I would rather live for the present and enjoy the things I can enjoy.

Life with a changing body

Multiple sclerosis frequently becomes visible at a time when other contemporaries, who are not affected, are in the prime of physical life. Physical malfunctions, whether conceived as medically minor or not, are thus set in the context of the expected present, and future development of 'normal' physical characteristics. Such 'normal' characteristics are themselves social constructs, and form a baseline against which people with multiple sclerosis measure their physical state, functioning, and performance. However, the sheer variety of physical symptoms and their functional effects which may arise in the course of the disease suggests that the subjective experience of bodily change is a complex process.

It may be hard to describe many of the bodily symptoms associated with multiple sclerosis; they 'do not fit neatly into a recognized "pigeon hole", and may seem odd to both the people who have them as well as those trying to help' (Burnfield 1985: 43).

Therefore understanding the relationships between deterioration in physical capacity and functional performance, and further, the meaning of this relationship in multiple sclerosis, is difficult. Deterioration may be variably spread over many bodily processes. Traditionally, in medical terms, the deterioration has been measured independently of the personal or social objectives of the person concerned, except where symptoms have proved too medically elusive to define – when they are likely to be medically ignored.

The difficulty of reconciling medical classifications of bodily symptoms in multiple sclerosis with the way they are perceived by those with the disease is posed by David. His descriptions of the way his legs and feet feel echo the rich texture of many accounts of individual symptoms, and the intrinsic complexity of their translation into medical terms (Monks 1986). After discussing his rather disaffected relations with doctors he notes their difficulties when they

ask how it feels. I say things like

'My feet feel as though they have been trampled.'
'The soles of my feet feel bruised most of the time.'
'It feels as though I've just had to run across a field of stinging nettles in bare feet.'

'It's like walking across a field of snow in Wellington boots without socks on.'

'Your leg feels as though you're wearing a tight elastic stocking.'

For some there is a general feeling of grief that taken-for-granted bodily health is gone for ever. Michelle experienced such a feeling but

> thought this feeling would pass but it hasn't. It gets worse with each attack. I feel that my body dies a bit more each time. It makes me much more aware of my mortality. I think my mental outlook would improve if I was to have a decent remission. . . . I just wish it [the disease] would leave me alone for a bit so I could think about something else for a change.

A disassociation from the body may begin to occur, and then become quite pronounced, as the physical effects of the disease are perceived as becoming dangerously destructive (Cassell 1976). Wright discusses this process in terms of what she calls a low 'self-connection gradient' (1983: 229). This gradient is a way of describing the extent to which any particular attribute, especially those related to the body, constitutes the core of the self. Is the real 'me' based on the appearance and performance of the body, deteriorating as it is, or is there a gradual disassociation of that real 'me' from the bodily decline? Janice indicates how she painfully seeks to explain and understand what is happening to her body with the development of multiple sclerosis:

> I hated my body at the time, I felt it had let me down by being inadequate, too weak to withstand living. I felt and still do a year later that this 'thing' which was taking over my body had nothing to do with 'me' inside it. I am trapped inside somewhere struggling to survive . . . [with that self] being used in the struggle to keep physically going each day. . . . Readjusting to seeing myself as disabled was initially very difficult, and still is hard each time some other part of my body is weakened.

It is subjectively impossible to sever the relationship between the body and the mind completely, whatever the extent of the disassociation between the inner self and that body (Birrer 1979). Sheila has been working through this problem:

At times I feel a completely different person who is doing all
the things I used to do. I feel more placid in many ways;
when I do get upset it has a devastating effect on me and I
feel ill for several days. Feeling ill can mean that all my
symptoms are more severe. I feel unreal at times almost as if
the real me had left my body and another person had entered
it. But I do not feel like the real me is looking on. The real
me is nowhere. I do not feel detached in any way. My body
feels so different, I think my mind is bound to be different
too, not just in what it thinks but in how it thinks. If my
body has to adjust to functioning with unprotected nerves then
so must the mind. Body and mind are irrevocably joined.

Contradictions in the interpretation of bodily appearance not
only may occur between the judgement of others and the judgement of self, but also may lie in the fragility of self-perception in
this situation. The struggle to maintain a positive self-image in
multiple sclerosis, particularly in the light of others' judgements
about the meaning of the body, is also difficult, as Sue indicates:

I was confused, I still felt fundamentally the same. My body
was different, I knew that all right, but inside it was me.
Normality is after all what you know. The male who is very
short is normal to himself, it is other people who make him
aware of an 'abnormality'. The 'ugly' female is 'normal' to
herself (try denying your own being), it's the others who
make her 'abnormal'. . . . On leaving hospital and finding the
mantle of 'disabled' placed firmly upon my unwilling
shoulders I entered a world which was alien, absurd and
ultimately defeating. My own grasp on my own identity was
no real match for the massed forces of society who firmly
believed themselves as 'normal' and myself just as firmly as
'abnormal'. I found myself inhabiting a stereotype. I became
my illness, I was only of interest because of it.

(quoted in Campling 1981: 47–8)

Urinary disturbances, described colloquially as incontinence –
which may affect up to a third of those with multiple sclerosis
(Beck, Warren, and Whitman 1981: 273) – are an area of
particular concern in relation to bodily performance. Associated,
as incontinence is, with the asexual world of the very young or
the very old, special efforts must be made to sustain a clear

identity with its onset. Although this symptom may be concealed or negotiated around in public – perhaps with difficulty – it cannot readily be hidden in intimate personal relationships. The distress with which the problem of incontinence can be regarded, especially in public, is indicated by Thelma:

> The worst thing about my MS is the problem I have with
> incontinence. It is utterly degrading to have to wear pads
> and to have to change them and not to know where the nearest
> loos are. Wearing summer clothes without tights makes it
> obvious that you are wearing it when you lie down.

The general fears of a demolished identity seem particularly embodied in the idea and the role of the wheelchair in the perceptions of those with multiple sclerosis. It is a socially visible representation of bodily decline. As with incontinence, the association with the inappropriate images of childhood and old age is hard to resist. The dependence which the wheelchair implies, and the anticipated ways in which being in a wheelchair restructures social relationships, may generate a fear of this status long before it materializes (I. Robinson, Lawson, and Wynne 1983: 10).

Janet indicates the potency of the image of the wheelchair, and all that it implies, in her thoughts:

> I was reeling [on discovering the diagnosis], especially as my
> image of MS was an horrific one based on the inevitability
> of degeneration – the wheelchair and worse. It has been this
> main aspect of coping with the disease which I have found
> most difficult to deal with. FEAR is the word!

Even for someone who sees her illness in a detached sort of way, the wheelchair image intrudes:

> I regard the illness quite clinically most of the time as I think
> it's interesting in a morbid sort of way. Now and then when
> I feel very bad . . . I get depressed as the threat of the
> wheelchair is hidden deep at the back of my mind still.

The decision to use a wheelchair, however fleetingly at first, appears to be as critical a point for some as the discovery of the diagnosis. It can be seen not only to represent an explicit mark of physical deterioration and increased dependence on others but also, even more important, to represent an implicit admission of the failure – or more positively a lack of success – of a personal strategy of resisting and thereby controlling the disease.

> When mentioning shops or museums, I can hear the word 'wheelchair' being suggested – this, I'm afraid, is my one blind spot. To me this is giving up my final independence and as long as I can walk, however shakily, I am not going to consider it.

The decision to use a wheelchair is not one that can easily be taken without a significant reassessment of personal goals and tactics, whatever the apparent functional benefits of using the wheelchair. It is the re-evaluation and re-establishment of these goals which constitute so much of the subjective experience of multiple sclerosis. Self-image and self-esteem depend on the capacity to do so effectively.

Self-image and self-esteem in multiple sclerosis

One of the earliest research findings on the psychological status of those with multiple sclerosis was the high incidence of what was described as euphoria. In 1922, for example, Brown and Davis's research indicated that the proportion of patients with euphoria was as high as 70 per cent. This finding was replicated by Cottrell and Wilson (1926) and became an established part of the repertory of symptoms assumed to be characteristic of multiple sclerosis. This 'typical' euphoric state suggested that patients' self-esteem and self-image was abnormally, indeed pathologically, positive. The concept of euphoria became seen as a major part of the core of an 'MS personality type'.

Later research has produced a far more complex perspective on the psychological status of those with the disease, with some researchers pointing out the substantial methodological problems associated with such studies (reviewed in Marsh, Ellison, and Strite 1983). The early research was undertaken using subjective clinical assessments of personality and mood where the definition, validity, and reliability of concepts such as 'euphoria' or 'depression' was found to be problematic by later writers. None the less the association of euphoria in multiple sclerosis has proved remarkably resilient.

In contrast to the earlier emphasis on euphoria, other research has indicated that depression is a significant concomitant of the disease (Goodstein and Ferrell 1977; F. A. Whitlock and Siskind 1980). In the latter study those with multiple sclerosis reported more episodes of depression than did other neurological patients. These findings have also been supported by the work of Baretz and Stephenson (1981) and Cleeland, Matthews, and Hopper (1970). However Matson and Brooks (1977) suggest that a positive self-image, and a low incidence of depression, is more typical of those with the disease.

The idea of a single 'MS personality', initially based on the widespread prevalence of euphoria, has also proved difficult to substantiate. More sophisticated analyses have indicated a diverse range of personality structures, linked with socio-cultural factors and with the stage of disease, in emotional responses to the illness (Gallineck and Kalinowsky 1958). Peyser, Edwards, and Poser's analysis of patients with multiple sclerosis on the Minnesota Multiphasic Personality Inventory (MMPI) yielded six distinctive clusters of personality traits. They state:

> We believe that past attempts to delineate a specific MS personality have failed for the reason that it would be naive to expect that all patients, regardless of their unique personal and symptom complex, will react in the same fashion and fit into a single pattern. Psychological adjustment should depend on the interplay of the nature and extent of involvement of the CNS [central nervous system], external variables and the patient's basic personality pattern.
>
> (Peyser, Edwards, and Poser 1980: 437)

In the light of these findings it is tempting to conclude that there is no recognizably distinct personality pattern implicated in multiple sclerosis, and that depression or euphoria, where they are found, are likely to be precipitated by events or situations not directly stemming from the disease process itself.

It appears that three kinds of arguable assumptions have guided much of the research into the disease. The first, as has been indicated, is that there must be some sort of single 'MS personality'. The second is made explicit by Whitlock. 'On common-sense grounds, it might be expected that patients with a progressively incapacitating disease with repeated remission and relapses would be depressed' (1984: 73). The third is that there is likely to be a positive correlation between degree of physical incapacity, depression, and low self-esteem.

Following Peyser, Edwards, and Poser's research the search for a single 'MS personality' type has slowed, although it is still the case that the second and third assumptions form the basis of much work on multiple sclerosis. Increasingly the evidence suggests that there is no clear relationship between physical incapacity and self-esteem. It is far more likely that situational determinants, individuals' past experiences, and reactions to them are critical in the way that self-esteem is generated and sustained.

Of the variety of diverse and conflicting findings in relation to self-esteem, the unexpected presence of a positive view of themselves and their lives, even by some of those who have substantial physical problems, is particularly interesting. Following earlier clinical findings this sort of response may still be characterized as 'euphoria', as in Schiffer, Rudick, and Herndon's account:

> [it is] a feeling of well being that is inappropriate to the reality of the situation and persists through time as more than merely mood fluctuation. There is a quality of anosognia, or indifference to disability in this state . . . it is often adaptive in the family system and is rarely a cause for complaint by either patient or family.
>
> (Schiffer, Rudick, and Herndon 1983: 314)

In this account the benchmark against which the 'euphoria' is measured is 'the reality of the situation', the implication being that this reality is not being defined appropriately by the patient and, in any case, requires a more circumspect – and less pathological – response. However, as they note such a positive outlook may be socially as well as personally adaptive. It is as much to this process of adaptation that researchers might look for an explanation of the phenomenon, as to the consequences of neurological or neuropsychological damage. As Sue puts it, 'denying your own being' (Campling 1981: 47–8), by adopting the stigmatizing judgements of others about the deterioration of one's body and capacities, may be less personally adaptive and 'realistic' than sustaining and reinforcing a positive image of that body and those capacities.

The genesis of such a positive view is shown in the account of Paula:

> That early diagnosis has changed the way I see myself. If I didn't know what was wrong with me, i.e. if I had to regard

myself as a fit person, I might be very dissatisfied. I can imagine asking, 'Why do I get so exhausted in hot weather? Why do my feet feel numb? Why do my legs tingle? What's wrong with my eye?' As a 'fit' person, I would be entitled to feel anxious and perplexed at all these peculiar things wrong with me.

As a person with MS, however, I see myself quite differently. Here I am with MS, yet I can walk, even run when the need arises! I can ride a bike, drive a car, cope with shopping, housework, and children, in fact live a normal life. I have MS, yet all I notice of it is a slight tingling, some numbness, and *slightly* blurred vision in one eye only. I feel very fortunate, and very grateful, to be only affected so mildly.

Such accounts should not be taken as representative of the 'typical' person with multiple sclerosis, but they do demonstrate the work that goes into extracting meaning out of illness. The positive view of life they record is not achieved easily; it does not come without struggle. It may have been wrested from the depths of depression; indeed it may be only a temporary interregnum and about the present rather than the future.

Depression and euphoria – begging their provenance for these purposes – may thus be the two faces of Janus. It may be as problematic to identify them as discrete and mutually exclusive categories, as it was argued to be in the case of 'denying', 'fighting', or 'accepting' the disease. In the struggle to create sense out of the illness, meaning is constructed dynamically. Depression may follow or precede euphoria, or both may coexist.

Coping, managing, adapting – the personal response to multiple sclerosis

The discussion in this chapter has led to two broad conclusions. First, that there is no simple relationship between physical disability and the subjective experience of multiple sclerosis. There is no evidence, for example, that those who are more functionally disabled have lower self-esteem. Second, there is little evidence that there is a common psychological pattern of adjustment to the disease. Attempts to demonstrate a general sequential pattern of response to multiple sclerosis from denial, through resistance, to acceptance, and integration have met with little success.

The weight of the existing evidence suggests that a diffuse combination of personal characteristics, the viability of personal and social relationships preceding the onset of the disease, and the nature and type of personal and social events occurring after the onset, are better predictors of adaptation or adjustment than the progress of the disease itself.

As Strauss has argued, 'the chief business of chronically ill persons is not just to stay alive or keep their symptoms under control, but to live as normally as possible despite the symptoms and the disease' (1984: 79).

Living as normally as possible is achieved through the negotiation of social relationships, and subjective perceptions of the self, as much as conditioned by the experience of the illness itself, its symptoms, and related functional problems.

Chapter four

Life with multiple sclerosis: social context and consequences

Being in a social world

By inference, much of the preceding discussion has indicated the significant role of social evaluations and behaviour in the experience of multiple sclerosis. The social context not only influences and constrains the options available to those with the disease, but also affects their perceptions of themselves. Just as significantly the physical, functional, and psychological manifestations of multiple sclerosis – or people's interpretations of them – feed into the social relationships of which those with the disease are a part. Burnfield describes this situation thus:

> MS . . . takes place in the universal cobweb of life. The strongest vibrations will be felt by those closest to the person who has the disease; but the effects of MS radiate beyond the immediate family and will make an impression and demand a response from friends, workmates and the community at large.
>
> (Burnfield 1985: 94)

The relationship between 'impression and response' which Burnfield notes does not of course take place in a virgin social world. Pre-existing beliefs about health and illness, about appropriate responses to changes in health, and more particularly about multiple sclerosis or its associated symptoms, condition the nature of the 'impression and response'. These beliefs are themselves related to social characteristics – such as age, sex, class – and by reference to 'normal' expectations of and about the behaviour and attitudes of the person concerned. Thus what Burnfield sees as the 'circle of ripples that is created as a stone [the event of multiple sclerosis] is dropped into a pond' (1985: 94) is even more complex than he suggests, for the pond itself reciprocally affects those ripples and their trajectory, often in an unpredictable way. Thus the negotiation of the meaning of multiple sclerosis is a continuing process.

Some of the strategies, through which negotiations over the social role of people who are deemed healthy or ill are conducted, have been explored in the work of the sociologists Goffman and Davis. Goffman (1963) developed the idea of 'passing', while Davis (1963) developed the idea of 'normalization'. If the concept of 'disassociation' (Miles 1979) is added to these two ideas, a useful analytical framework is provided which can be applied to the interpretation of the social strategies of people with multiple sclerosis. 'Passing' can be described as the strategy of passing oneself off as not having a disease or disability by attempting to maintain its social invisibility. 'Normalization' can be described as a strategy whereby, despite socially visible signs of the condition, a determined attempt is made to carry on life as normal, in which the disease is a part of that normal life, but not the dominant part. 'Disassociation' can be described as a strategy where a separate and 'disease-based' life-style is developed, where the primary reference group for beliefs and behaviour is that of others with the disease, rather than the community at large. Two studies which have sought to use and develop these three categories are those of Cunningham (1977) and Miles (1979).

The strategy of 'passing' is available to many in the early stages of multiple sclerosis. Cunningham indicates how people with the disease redesign their social lives, often with the aid of a 'collaborator' – perhaps a close family member – so that any physical malfunction is concealed or acceptably explained (1977: 51–2). Indeed without that 'collaborator' providing support or a social alibi, the strategy is hard to pursue successfully. A stay in hospital for example may be plausibly covered by reference to a brief holiday, or problems of mobility may be concealed by restructuring exactly how and when others see movement from one place to another. At a different level

one woman, when asked by a stranger what was wrong with her foot (she was limping badly and had an unsteady gait) claimed that she had sprained her ankle. A man who works as an architect claimed he needed new glasses rather than

acknowledge to his colleagues that he had multiple sclerosis
and was suffering from impaired vision.

(Cunningham 1977: 51)

This technique of passing may be used, but it is a socially
dangerous strategy requiring constant alertness, quick thinking,
and foresight. Being 'found out' is a continual concern. In
Goffman's analysis such people may be termed as 'discreditable'
(1963) – capable of being discredited. They hold a potentially
stigmatizing secret, which if it was revealed might damage their
relationships with others. Elizabeth talks about her secret:

> I feel changed by it, that I'm different in a crowd – as yet my
> disabilities don't show and only I know about them.
> Sometimes when I'm amongst people who don't know me I'm
> aware of this 'secret knowledge' – I'm not perfect anymore.

'Passing' may place a considerable burden on the 'collaborator',
whose complicity may be unwillingly gained and retained. Thus
there is a double burden, on those 'collaborators' who know 'the
truth', and on the person with multiple sclerosis to maintain their
'fictional' identity as a person with no disability. Danny's wife, for
example, found her burden something she could not sustain:

> Danny made a decision that I felt was wrong but it was his
> decision. He decided to keep the diagnosis secret. I think he
> somehow felt guilty about it; I don't know why. As well he
> feared people would pity him and treat him differently if they
> knew. Gradually life returned to normal [after the attack which
> led to his diagnosis]. Danny went back to work and we never
> mentioned MS. The secret weighed heavily on me at times
> and I confided in a few close friends. I felt that I was
> betraying Danny by telling people.

It does appear that the cost of 'collaboration' in 'passing' in these
circumstances is high. Spouses especially may feel they themselves
have little to gain from such a strategy, which may deprive them
of open access to other close family members as well as to those
outside the family circle. Given these problems such a strategy is
used with regularity only where stakes are high. Such a situation
occurs where there is a fear that employment may be jeopardized
by common knowledge of the condition; this issue is discussed
later in this chapter.

As a postscript to this discussion of 'passing' it is important to point out that there are others with multiple sclerosis who find that they can pass for normal when they would not wish to do so. In managing uncertainty the difficulty of persuading others of the credibility of 'invisible' symptoms like fatigue and incontinence was noted. Paradoxically, on the one hand there are those who conceal their symptoms to avoid social recognition of their illness, and, on the other hand, those who seek to gain social recognition as sick people and cannot because their symptoms are socially elusive.

Realistically, however, many people with multiple sclerosis are faced with the strategy of 'normalizing' their disease either because of their highly visible functional problems, or because they seek to reduce the discrepancy between their own and others' perceptions of themselves. In Miles's study 'normalizing' was one of the two major strategies adopted by people with the disease. There was an attempt to treat the disease as a visible and accepted component of social life, but one that did not dominate social interaction. The clear reference group was the community of the healthy rather than the community of the sick (1979: 323–5).

Sustaining this view of the disease may be difficult unless 'deviance disavowal' can be accomplished (Davis 1961). Such 'deviance disavowal' in the case of multiple sclerosis first involves breaking the mould of others' stereotypical views of the disease, re-establishing a 'normal' identity, and then sustaining that identity. But it is clear that this is a process, not a single event. Constant negotiation is required, particularly where social interactions frequently involve strangers. Each new interaction becomes a new negotiation, a negotiation which involves time, effort, and commitment. David, for example, indicates the problems raised by his moving house:

I have had more difficulties in general because of my moves. . . . Lack of continuity itself is an intrusive and often unpleasant fact. What I mean is this for example. When I met my next-door neighbours, the husband said to me, 'Have you always had this or what?'

In fact, I've only known that I had it for a couple of years, and only had real difficulty in walking for half that time, and before then I was more active, a better sports player, and better co-ordinated than most. Almost no one, except my family, has known me before and after.

He is particularly concerned that the stereotypical view of him eliminates his past. It is as though the power of the stereotype has wiped away all his previous achievements.

One of the problems in this strategy of 'normalization' is to allow the symptoms and the illness to be brought to the attention of others, but to have them rejected as the defining characteristic. Strauss gives an example of such a strategy in a young woman with multiple sclerosis:

> She brings your focus smack down on her abnormality underlining it . . at . . . one and the same time addressing you in a manner commensurate with young professional women who are actively involved in interesting jobs and doing it well, and at the same time making you address yourself to the very aspect of her which places all other aspects suspect or in question.
>
> (Strauss 1984: 82)

In this case one of the problems is not to let the symptoms so flood the interaction that it proves virtually impossible to treat them as merely a marginal intrusion in the relationship. As Miles points out the credibility of the strategy – she calls it a major weakness – depends on the availability and willingness of healthy others to reinforce it and enter into normalized interaction (1979: 324). Roger seems confident that they will do so although he has to make some concessions:

> I never hid from anyone what I had – my attitude was if they know then they won't keep saying, 'What's the matter with your leg?' I don't want sympathy or anyone to feel sorry for me. I have a positive attitude to this – I can and I will with certain reservations. Lots of things I can do – some things I can't. So what – some able-bodied people have their failings – why not me.

On the other hand it is clear that Maria is having major difficulties when she 'comes out' in public with her disease. She feels that the absence of a socially available stereotype of multiple sclerosis leads to the imputation of even more stigmatizing behaviour:

> My own situation is very complex – [people round here] have

an inborn dread of the disease and only in the past few
months have I come out into the open and said what I have.
Nobody here has heard of MS, let alone knows anyone who
has it. I live in a small town and everyone knows that there
is something wrong – they probably think I am drunk from
morning to night.

In Miles's study there was no evidence that the strategy of
normalization was automatically undermined by increasing
physical disability. The viability of the strategy depended far more
on the personal and social characteristics and context of those
negotiating the meaning of the disease. None the less, the greater
the degree of physical disability, the more the effort it may require
to sustain a 'normal' identity. This is particularly the case with
those who use wheelchairs, who may be constrained by social
imagery generally antithetical to such an identity. However, as
Joe shows such problems may be confronted head on. As part of
his philosophy of life, he dealt with an unpleasant comment with
something of a social *tour de force*:

> One day [at work] Colin called me a smelly cripple – only in
> a joking manner. I was taken a bit aback at first, but thought
> that didn't hurt so went over to the . . . intercom and broadcast
> to all . . . that Colin, and I described him, had called me, a
> poor invalid in a wheelchair, a smelly cripple. Poor old Colin,
> who was really a nice guy, was so embarrassed he didn't
> know where to put his face. So I introduced this phraseology
> into my vocabulary; now a lot of people call me this. Even
> my mate Raymond, who figures a lot in what I have done,
> calls me a Raspberry Ripple (rhyming slang for smelly
> cripple). Please, please don't get me wrong, I don't say that
> everyone who is disabled should be called a smelly cripple.
> I'm just saying that as far as I'm concerned the word cripple
> doesn't hurt me now, and what I am trying to say to anyone
> else in the same boat, don't be afraid of nothing, if you believe
> in something stand up and be counted.

Michael found what he deemed to be much more accepting attitudes enabling him to sustain his identity with rather less effort:

> I was on the station [in my wheelchair] waiting for my train
> to be indicated when identical twin girls came straight up to
> me. One said, 'Why are you sitting in that pram?' I tried to

explain that my legs didn't work very well. They were right little chatter-boxes. They were going to Granny at Plymouth and wouldn't get there until the middle of the night. Before long they had climbed up one on each knee – then mum turned round. 'Oh,' she said, 'You've found a new friend have you. Send them away if they are a nuisance to you' and carried on talking with her husband. If we are talking about attitudes towards disabled people . . . you beat that.

Miles did find, however, that the majority of her study group engaged in the third strategy, that is what she calls a strategy of disassociation, what Cunningham calls 'withdrawal' (1977: 55). In essence life was redesigned around the community of those with multiple sclerosis. They became the prime social reference group. In part this was determined by the range of ordinary social activities now no longer possible. However, a more important factor in both Cunningham and Miles's studies was the increasingly difficult relationship between people with the disease, and others. In brief this group with multiple sclerosis felt stigmatized. Miles expresses it thus:

> [They felt] that healthy people did not understand their feelings and problems but pitied them and felt embarrassed in their presence; that past relationships had ended in disappointment and bitterness and the best policy was to keep away. They regarded the illness as being of overwhelming importance in their lives and described their social situation as changed and inferior.
>
> (Miles 1979: 324)

One of the key aspects of this process was the degree to which a relatively fragile positive self-image was protected by the reduction of contacts with others with little knowledge of the disease. Social safety was found either with other people with multiple sclerosis, or by reducing all social contacts to a minimum.

Miles notes that the couples in her study agreed on their strategy. That is those whose spouses with the disease sought to disengage themselves from 'normal' social contacts also felt the same way. However this view is increasingly suspect. It suggests a high and uniform congruence of interests between spouses on this issue, on which the literature on the role of carers casts doubts (see for example Briggs and Oliver 1985), and on which there is more specific evidence which conflicts with Miles's observations (for example Robinson 1988). The fact that couples adopted the behaviour appropriate to the strategy of 'disassociation' does not necessarily imply their individual support for it. An illustration of some of the possible problems comes from the comments of Marjorie, whose husband after an attack of the disease had virtually exclusive contacts with others with multiple sclerosis:

> At this time [when her husband was badly affected] I felt completely overtaken by MS. I saw it, spoke it, lived it, hated it, all day, everyday. Any outside contact was MS; any visitor was to see Walter and see how his MS was. . . . I wish we could meet more people without MS, but because of Walter, or anyone with a disability, it is more or less impossible. Only other MS sufferers know how each other feels.

In this case and others the term 'identity spread' (Strauss 1984: 81) can be used to describe the way the effects, indeed the stigma of the disease, come to circumscribe a family unit, not just the individual with multiple sclerosis. As Burnfield puts it, 'When one person in the family has MS, then the whole family "has MS" as well' (1985: 95).

The strategy of disassociation seems to lead to a greater likelihood of this 'identity spread' happening than in the other strategies.

In concluding this section it would be wrong to assume that passing, normalizing, and disassociation are mutually exclusive categories, or that there is some inexorable progression from one to the other. On the contrary both Miles and Cunningham indicate, in spite of this categorization in their research, that people's strategies are often fluid, and their success not guaranteed. At different times and in different social settings all three strategies may be deployed.

The future of relationships: coming to terms with multiple sclerosis

As a major component of the social world, within which the disease unfolds, close social relationships with friends, partners, spouses, and families form a very considerable component of the experience of multiple sclerosis. The analytical difficulty is to attempt to distinguish the specific effects of the condition, and its interpretation, from the 'normal' multiplicity of factors which affect such relationships. In the complex interior of intimate relationships any such distinction may be arbitrary and inappropriate. However, some themes and patterns emerge from the study of those relationships which do indicate the part that experience of the disease plays in them.

At a general level, knowledge of the disease itself may 'disable the normal', as Blaxter puts it (1976: 202). That is this knowledge immediately places relationships with persons with multiple sclerosis outside the pale of the normal. In this context the critical period of risk to relationships, in the very early stages of a disability involving one of the partners, has been noted by both Sainsbury (1970) and Blaxter (1976). In multiple sclerosis those relationships may be seen as embodying a socially disabling core (Gorman, Rudd, and Ebers 1984: 219). However, it would be an error to see the knowledge of the diagnosis as introducing a common, uniform, and negative element in close relationships. Responses may be complex, affected as they are by many other factors. For some the effect is indeed negative. For example Lucy's own immediate reaction to her diagnosis was to see her future relationships as irreparably damaged:

> I had to reappraise my career prospects . . . and I was upset
> at the thought of perhaps having to give up my independence
> . . . [but] my main reaction was that I would never get married
> now – I thought that even if someone wanted me, I might
> be too much of a burden on them.

The future of relationships already established may also be under severe and immediate threat as in Justine's case. Her account demonstrates the way the diagnostic information precipitated a whole series of threatening events to her intending marriage; the extent to which it crystallized an array of potent and conflicting attitudes, and the difficult position in which she now finds herself:

> Arthur [her boyfriend] was not happy with it all [her MS and
> being in hospital]. His parents had said that he should finish
> with me while we still had not married. Arthur was obviously
> in quite a turmoil and went to see Dr Y [her neurologist]
> and my parents. Dr Y was apparently very sympathetic
> towards Arthur but was unable to give him any reassuring

'She'll probably be all right in the end'. So when I returned home to my parents . . . Arthur told me that he thought it would be best for us to finish. I was stunned. This was now for me all-out survival . . . so I simply said to Arthur that if he finished with me I would commit suicide – I honestly didn't care. I think that I would have done. I went from one extreme to the other and then started to plead with Arthur. Was it my fault I was like this? Why shouldn't he adapt? I was furious as well as hurt. I could not run away from the disease, he could. I told him I thought he was pathetic. In the end he told me that he would give it three years. If after that time I had not got any worse, then we'd get married. Four years later we're both single and I've got this death sentence hanging over me – if I have another attack he'll finish with me. Not very pleasant.

For relationships apparently already in a fragile state for other reasons, the knowledge of the diagnosis may trigger major decisions, as in Barbie's vigorous and tough response to her husband:

Straight after being told [the diagnosis] I went to work because I couldn't stand being with my husband who was crying. To cut a long story short, my husband couldn't cope. He used to sit with his head in his hands saying, 'What am I going to do when you are in a wheelchair'. I tried to point out to him that I am one of the lucky ones; I am not yet in a wheelchair and hopefully never will be as I have only a mild case of MS. . . . The decision to leave my husband came when my best friend had a baby. . . . I had always wanted to have children and with my husband being the way he was I knew I could never have his children.

Other relationships may be cemented rather than undermined by the discovery of the diagnosis. This appears to be the case where the partner without the disease has some other characteristic which itself might be construed as potentially 'disabling'. In the case of Brenda her age was that 'disabling' component:

[After her engagement] we married the following year after much discussion – he was prepared to take on someone ten years older than him and I was prepared for his MS. . . . [Although] I have found it restricting after years of freedom and pleasing myself, on the other hand I am at least in the position of knowing what I was taking on – and not having MS foisted on me – like he had – or many wives.

Unlike Brenda whose continuation in and positive view of the future of her relationship was conditioned by the thought of mutual support, Clive sees his decision to keep his marriage going, following the diagnosis, as entirely a sacrifice on his part:

I had reached the point where I was thinking of leaving. I would have been worse off financially but I would have had time to myself. I had planned to move in with two colleagues when the diagnosis of MS arrived. Much self-analysis followed, resulting in the decision that I couldn't leave, that my obligations were so great that I had to stay. Leaving in the previous situation would have caused pain but I had decided that this was more than balanced by the eventual improvement in everyone's situation. MS just tipped the scales the other way. The thought of her [his wife] becoming incapacitated and the family being broken up was a possibility that I felt I had to prevent.

The process of marital readjustment immediately following the diagnosis can be an extremely difficult one, as has already been implied. After some of these difficulties have been worked through, a more reflective view can be taken of what in retrospect can be seen to have been a very traumatic time. For example, Marcia says:

My overall reaction was not good. I think I felt I had to do as much as possible in a short time so I started doing things which were quite unlike me, and caused lots of problems for my husband. For example I stayed out a lot with friends, and started drinking after work. I went to parties and dances without my husband. I even stayed out all night a couple of times. None of these things I had done before and I generally spent a year thinking and feeling sorry for myself. I also decided that my husband and my four sons depended on me too much and decided they would be better learning to do without me. So without realizing what I was doing I cut myself off from them. . . . I now realize that I am capable of continuing as I am and may never become disabled so I am back to my normal self.

Terry's wife discovered her husband had been planning a dramatic end to their relationship on hearing the diagnosis:

It took me months to accept the new reality [after the diagnosis]. I cannot express what went through my mind in these few months. I can imagine how Terry did suffer! Later he confessed that all sorts of things went through his mind. He even thought of committing suicide so that I could start a new life with someone else. He wanted to spare our daughter and myself from a troublesome life with him. But fortunately he has been strong enough to overcome the crisis and little by little he started reconciling himself to his new condition. I do admire him for his courage and strength.

As Blaxter indicates in her study (1976: 206), it is the marriages and relationships of younger people at the onset of the impairment who appear to be most vulnerable to difficulties and breakdown, and for whom referral for support or help was far less likely.

Living together: change and continuity

The reordering of relationships which is part of the process of living with multiple sclerosis is a continuing process. At one level it is conditioned by the likelihood of constantly changing functional problems; at another by the 'ordinary' life changes anticipated by young adults, and at another in the re-evaluation of future goals or possibilities as a result of both of these sets of changes.

Strauss sees the major problems as lying in the constant redefinition of normality in such relationships as the levels of functioning get worse. This can result in greater and greater commitments by family, relatives, and friends, and he notes:

When friends or relatives will not enter into more and more onerous arrangements, necessitated by lower levels of functioning then they in turn opt out – by divorce, separation or abandonment. Those who are ill from multiple sclerosis or other severe forms of neurological illness . . . are likely to face this kind of abandonment from others.

(Strauss 1984: 86)

However the evidence to support this observation is insubstantial. Although specific divorce rates may be higher amongst people with the disease (I. Robinson, Lawson, and Bakes 1983) there is little data, as yet, to indicate that these rates are closely related to the degree of functional disability. On the contrary, as was noted in the previous section, the weight of the evidence suggests that marital breakdowns, separations, and divorces tend to occur earlier in the course of the disease, when serious, constant, and permanent functional problems are in the minority. This is not to say that severe functional problems do not have a profound effect on relationships – they plainly do – but that the response to those effects in themselves is perhaps less likely to be abandonment, separation, or divorce, than earlier in the course of the disease.

A particular area of difficulty which does arise in relationships, into which multiple sclerosis intrudes, is in the reconfiguration of what might be called the social roles of the parties to the relationship. Such roles which embrace the relative status and power of those in the relationship, as well as the specific duties and obligations they have, are subject to negotiation. They are also affected by functional capacities, and by the expectations and constraints of others outside the relationship itself. Dependency is a useful organizing idea in relation to which the issue of social roles can be discussed.

Of course the value attached to independence, and the fear of dependence, is embodied in general cultural values:

independence . . . goes along with ability, masculinity, leadership and rugged individualism. To be independent is reassuring that one will be able to take care of oneself and not be dependent on the uncertain solicitude of others. Dependence on the other hand is often disvalued. It is associated with weakness, femininity, indecision, selfishness and helplessness.

(Wright 1983: 405–6)

Wright goes on to argue that the cultural antithesis between the two states creates particular dilemmas for disabled people, or those who fear disablement, because of the invariably negative and stigmatizing way in which dependence is considered. It is not surprising therefore that those with multiple sclerosis and their families should pay such attention to the possibility and effects of dependence.

In her study of people with multiple sclerosis Cunningham uses the notion of dependence to delineate ways in which social roles within family relationships may be modified, and in which conflict and problems may be generated (1977: 59–63). As she indicates, the issue of increasing dependence has a whole series of parameters, physical, psychological, and financial (1977: 59).

At a practical level dependence implies reliance on others for the accomplishment of day-to-day tasks. Social roles within a family setting may be quickly changed, as tasks which were previously undertaken personally become difficult without the presence, time, and co-operation of others. At one extreme, with very severe functional impairment virtually everything may require the complete attention of others, as in Raymond's case:

> During the last two years my wife's condition has deteriorated to the extent that I now have to wash and dress her every morning, get her downstairs, feed her, bath her, assist her with toilet functions – she is now catheterized.
>
> You will see from my comments . . . that I am now nursemaid, cook, companion, and provider for her daily needs although the two friends do the household cleaning and ironing for me. . . .
>
> It is true to say that life has become extremely routine from what it used to be, and the stress of trying to look after my wife has begun to take its toll.

A number of important points are raised here. The physical dependency produced not only has led to a complete restructuring of social roles, but also has perhaps even more importantly undermined the sense of reciprocal value in the relationship. It is as though the marriage operates with the shadow of Raymond's wife. She has lost control of her body and her sexuality, and he has become a constant and intimate body 'maintenance man'. In the process both of them appear to be struggling – not very successfully – to sustain their essential selves independently to the crumbling physical shell of her body. Both Raymond and his wife are prisoners of this problem, in which the continuous and undifferentiated routine indeed seems equivalent to 'serving time' – perhaps even a life sentence. As his physical capacities become greater relative to hers, his choices have become as limited as those of his wife. Despite the evident difficulties of the situation – perhaps because of them – Raymond and many others continue doggedly in the face of very considerable adversity.

There are of course relationships in which managing severe functional problems in the family home setting proves impossible.

It is not necessarily functional problems alone, however, that determine whether an institutional solution is sought and obtained. Kay expresses a whole range of emotions – anger, regret, bitterness, grief, sorrow – about when her husband went into a Home. She is now having to work out how to come to terms with this:

> I thought he [her husband] only went into the Home on an assessment basis for one month [three years ago], but when I called to collect him I was informed by the Matron that she had no intention of releasing him into my care as he was better in the Home. There was no reaction from my husband when he was asked if he would like to go home with me or stay where he was. I was absolutely stunned and I am afraid I just walked out and drove away. . . . I was bitterly opposed to my husband going into the Home, and felt that somehow I had let him down but he was becoming increasingly difficult to manage both physically and temperamentally. Although he was walking with the aid of a frame when he went into the Home the residents are soon confined to a wheelchair all day, and catheterized so that the staff are not bothered too much. . . . I sometimes think he does not know me anymore and he certainly does not know our son. . . . I have been deeply affected mentally and physically by this chain of events and feel my husband did nothing to help himself. . . . I regret having to say this, but if I had known what was in front of me those many years ago when we got married I would have turned in the opposite direction; I would never encourage marriage between two people one of whom is handicapped with no chance of recovery. The burden is intolerable.

Even in this situation where the functional and other problems precipitated by multiple sclerosis appeared to trigger the journey to the Home, it is not clear to what extent pre-existing difficulties in the relationship compounded both the event and its after-effects.

The majority of those with multiple sclerosis, and those in close relationships with them, are not likely to face such intractable functional problems as Raymond, Kay, and their spouses had to confront. However, in considering situations where there is less functional impairment, and therefore technically less dependence on others, different problems are presented. They may prove paradoxically to be as hard to manage as where that functional impairment is very severe.

One of the major problems is the joint negotiation of the meaning and effects of multiple sclerosis – particularly in relation to the dependence it implies. Strauss indicates that the perception of the trajectory of the illness may be quite different between wives and husbands, friends and relatives. Cunningham found that wives and husbands of people with the disease tended to judge them as less capable of performing tasks, than those people judged themselves to be (1977: 60–3; see also Lincoln 1981 and Robinson 1988; for a contrary view see Radford and Trew 1987: 129). This generally found discrepancy itself has considerable consequences not only for the negotiated redistribution of specific tasks, but also more broadly for wider social roles, and for the idea of 'partnership', 'equality', or 'worth' in the relationship. Judgements about the ability to perform tasks imply judgements about dependence and independence, and go to the core of who and what people are.

The negotiation in the early stages of the disease is often complicated by relapses and remissions which fail to provide a stable and predictable basis on which to work out the relationship. Does the negotiation proceed on current 'capacities' whatever they are, or on assumptions of the best possible or worst possible case? Of course the judgement of capacities themselves, as has been indicated, is both subjective and likely to be heavily influenced by factors unrelated to the disease.

Some with the disease feel that they have to battle to sustain their worth at all, even with little current physical impairment:

On my diagnosis, and before, my husband's way of coping with the crisis was to take over, which I was sometimes quite happy for him to do, but this (a) gave *him* no time or space to grieve and sort things out for himself and (b) in the long run would have made me a less and less effective parent and member of the family group. So it was quite a slog to re-establish our relative positions in the group, and it took me quite a time to be in a position to comfort *him*.

Marion has spent much time thinking through her relationship with her husband and believes she has now resolved the question of their mutual respect for each other's role:

I strongly feel that disability is always far worse for the onlooker, especially for the spouse than the person going through it. I remember very recently being in tears when, after a long walk, my . . . old dog could not easily get to her feet, and I instantly thought, if this is how I feel about the dog, how much worse Tim will feel watching me. . . . He says he felt very unsure what to do as he felt that no matter how encouraging he tried to be, he could never tell how I was reacting. There were, and are, times when he offers a down-to-earth approach when I might be in need of particular understanding. On another occasion he tried to offer me sympathy and I told him to stop 'fussing'. With hindsight, I can see how difficult I must have been to live with; on the surface, I appeared to be coping very well, showing a positive stiff-upper-lip attitude, whereas I often needed tremendous reassurance. I always did, and do, minimize the difficulties I have, trying not to cause unnecessary worry. . . . [However] I have found that hiding one's true feelings can lead to complete misunderstandings . . . with truth, honesty, and togetherness, I feel we shall overcome whatever the future holds.

The mental or physical struggle by people with the disease to maintain independence, to continue to accomplish all or most of the tasks they did before – especially when functional problems become greater – produces ambivalent responses. On the one hand such a spirited approach may be considered positively as a manifestation of their inner determination to overcome the condition, but also be considered negatively as being at the personal and emotional expense of others in the relationship (Locker 1983: 147–9). The traditional rehabilitation approach to chronic disease, with its emphasis on assumed family unity in supporting the needs of 'the patient', may completely fail to recognize the existence of such a dilemma, and the potentially serious conflicts to which it gives rise. For example, Power in his study of the family setting in multiple sclerosis argues that

A family was considered adjusted if the family members showed positive coping strategies and reorientated their lives to encompass new illness-related events, such as transporting the ill spouse to the clinic for twice weekly visits, assisting the patient to move safely round the house when mobility was severely limited, changing the frequency of social activities when the family budget was reduced, and the willingness of the spouse or children to find part-time employment to compensate for financial deficits due to the patient's unemployment. Added criteria for positive adjustment revolved around the family's description of their 'normal' family life, and their conviction that this customary functioning had not been seriously disrupted because of the diagnosis of multiple sclerosis.

(Power 1985: 79)

By this account any strategy other than wholehearted support for the needs of the person with multiple sclerosis is deemed a maladjustment of the *family*. Third-party interventions based on such a view may in themselves destabilize the delicately negotiated fabric of family adaptation.

Some of the dilemmas of families working out how best to deal with the problems of the disease are shown in this struggle over the issue of mobility:

I found it very hard (and still do!) to watch George struggling to do something for himself when I could easily do it for him, but I do not want to feel later that I took his independence from him. His increasing independence has to be 'voluntary', so to speak. Sometimes however my own emotional needs demand that I take action if I am to avoid feeling martyred.

(Christine, quoted in Briggs and Oliver 1985: 38)

For those in a caring role then – however close their relationship – incapacity may be easier to cope with than marginal capacity. This may explain in part the findings of Cunningham and others, mentioned above, about the perception of functional capacity by spouses of their partners with the disease. Elizabeth makes the issue very explicit:

When I am tired I cannot cope with helping him walk and encourage him to use his wheelchair – which is the worst possible thing for him, and, of course, makes me feel guilty.

One of the most difficult periods of my life was last summer when Robert got flu. The *easy* part was when he was totally paralysed and had to stay in bed. The difficulties began when he wanted to get up, couldn't do it himself, and I wasn't strong enough to help. It gave me a shock to find that I couldn't get regular nursing help, so once again I had to rely on the neighbours to help me lift Robert. They don't mind, but I find it difficult not to be independent.

However, it is important to note that the burden of caring in a relationship, is not only – perhaps not even primarily – one of physical management. It is a burden of the knowledge of the fundamental personal and social effects of multiple sclerosis on a relationship. Such a knowledge influences Clive's view of the future:

> I have grown more distant from my wife and children. We accept that we do little together. . . . [However] our marriage, or at least my attitude towards it, has settled down. I accept my responsibility to Donna to care for her if her MS becomes a handicap. . . . I see the last ten years of my life as a failure. I have achieved nothing for myself. . . . I now feel I can achieve something worthwhile . . . yet I see supporting Donna as an indispensable part of this. . . . Donna's illness at the moment requires no action on my part, since it in no way disables her. However the increased possibility of disablement has brought about far-reaching consequences on our marriage and myself.

There is a multiplicity of patterns of response evident in relationships into which multiple sclerosis is interpolated. This is not surprising as multiple sclerosis is merely one dimension in a considerable array of dimensions which constitute and affect relationships. However, multiple sclerosis, and its actual, perceived, and anticipated effects, often acts as catalyst, trigger, or precipitator for outcomes to relationships.

Parents and children

Concerns about children occupy the thoughts of many of those in relationships restructured by multiple sclerosis – as they do in other relationships. Decisions as to whether, when, or how many children to have, and how best to care for them, are of particular moment. The special potency of such decisions in the context of the disease is based on a number of considerations, functional, social, psychological, and symbolic.

At one level there has been much debate about the effect that pregnancy and childbirth have on the course of the disease, whether indeed they may trigger onset, or exacerbations, or in some other way accelerate deterioration. The formal evidence on this point seems at present to be generally inconclusive. However there is some indication that the number of relapses may be greater in the post-partum period than in women who have not been pregnant, and that pregnancy may, in certain circumstances, precipitate the disease in those already with 'premorbid' multiple sclerosis (Leibowitz *et al.* 1967). However, more recent reviews of the evidence suggest a far more benign role for pregnancy in the course of multiple sclerosis (Matthews 1985: 85–7). The nature of the debate may itself result in conflicting advice about the advisability of pregnancy in those with the disease; advice which, on the evidence of pregnant women with other disabilities, may be as influenced by views about disabled mothers, as about the disease itself (National Childbirth Trust 1984: 11–12). As the onset of the disease is, in any case, highly probable at the time of maximum fertility, such points are likely to confront many people with the disease and their partners.

Decisions about pregnancy raise a series of significant considerations in the presence of multiple sclerosis. Such decisions may focus attention on the future; the potentially or actually declining body; the stability and strength of relationships; sexuality; motherhood and fatherhood; mortality; the expectations and response of others; and the likelihood of children themselves contracting the disease. In this sense decisions to have children involve confronting a series of major social and psychological issues, particularly for women, which may relegate those relating to the physiological effects alone to a relatively minor role.

The decision as to whether to have a child or not – as well as reflections after such a decision – features extensively in accounts of those with the disease. Tricia says:

> We've [herself and her husband] had to come to terms with having no children and this was tricky for me and sometimes still can be. But we don't think we can take the risk of having a baby and possibly Ralph [her husband] having to cope with that and a badly disabled wife.

Chris has been thinking through the same issue in relation to her boyfriend:

I doubt that we will have children as I feel they would not have a fair chance and Rob doesn't feel he could deal with it. He often finds the dog enough to deal with, but that can apply to me too. Anyway I think he is too harsh on himself, but who knows whether it would be a good idea for us to have children.

On the other hand Claire became pregnant again against medical advice and did not regret it:

Everytime I went to outpatients [for check-ups after her diagnosis] I told them I wanted to have children but they advised me against it. . . . It took exactly one year to get pregnant again [after her miscarriage] and we were so pleased and happy. By this time the doctors had given up advising me not to have children. Everything was great with the pregnancy; I felt marvellous for nine months . . . and had our little girl. . . . I'm so proud of her, she fulfilled our lives. . . . I feel that he [her husband] has got a lot to put up with; I feel sorry for him. . . . I realize that a lot of partners can't cope with the responsibility; I'm lucky but I'd like to think I'd do the same in reverse.

Megan expresses her regrets:

I regret not having a daughter; I always wanted a daughter, but I've got some godchildren and a niece. We both thought it best not to put any extra strain on what there is to do already, by having children to look after.

Being a mother, or being a father, looking after children, and bringing them up raises a further set of issues. One of these is how, when, and what to tell the children about the disease. Sally feels relaxed about the way that her children have responded to this information:

The kids have been quite matter of fact about my illness. My sons ask about it now and again whilst I don't believe they worry about it a lot (as I have never had any debilitating symptoms at all), they are open and up-front enough to talk about it when they feel like it, and I don't push it. They know as much as I do about my prognosis, and that they are not likely to catch/have it in their genes.

Of course the circumstances in which information about the

disease is imparted to children may be unanticipated and be far from ideal.

On Christmas Eve 1980 Gordon had an attack . . . he was literally crawling around the house. . . . We were both upset and frightened. We felt we couldn't tell the children there and then we never thought of a doctor. . . . Gordon was trying to pretend that all was well for the children's sake, yet he was very irritable . . . [then he went to hospital]. . . . He was very down [in hospital] and I spent a lot of time with him. I was staying with his mother and I had the children with me, but Gordon demanded so much of my time that I had to send the children to my mother. . . . I was very sad parting with them. Gordon was eventually discharged from hospital to his mother's house. . . . I was anxious to be reunited with the kids, and becoming impatient with Gordon because he did not feel able to go home. I came home without him.

Adapting to a condition like multiple sclerosis and to parenthood is not an easy task. Abby, in reflecting on her role as mother, feels guilty, concerned, and ultimately cheated in bringing up her children:

Looking back the biggest problem I had to cope with was the children. Small children are exhausting at the best of times. The winters seem worst because of all the illnesses they get. I seem to feel worse when they are ill even when I don't catch the same bug and when we are all ill together it is hell because I am the one who has to keep going and has no chance of retiring to bed.

I cannot say that I enjoyed their early childhood but it is hardly their fault. When I was well and rested life was quite pleasant, but that didn't happen too often. I longed for the time when they were at school full-time but felt guilty about wishing their childhood away. There were times when I felt that they were making my condition worse, particularly when their behaviour was trying or difficult. I get so irritable and my patience is limited when I feel ill. I just pray that my all-too-frequent outbursts when they were small have not harmed them.

There have been times when I have felt cheated. I had imagined enjoying my babies.

Abby emphasizes her concern with her own moods and needs in this situation as much as the physical problems she faced. Georgina's account, on the other hand, is a triumphant view of how she overcame considerable physical difficulties in managing her baby.

[Neighbours, her mother, and her husband had looked after her three children after a very lengthy period in hospital during an attack which left her paralysed from the waist down.] I continued to go daily for my physiotherapy and neighbours collected Margaret and Rachel from nursery school. Barbara came with me in her carry-cot. I couldn't lift her but we managed anyway. In the morning George used to take Barbara out of her cot and put her in her pram in the hall downstairs. When I was dressed and had slid myself down the stairs on my bottom, I would wedge myself between the zimmer [walking frame] and the high pram. There I would wash and change the baby then feed her etc. We had a wooden plank with a blanket wrapped round it which I propped against the side of the pram and slid her down the plank and on to the floor, where she was able to roll and kick until I rolled her back up the plank into the pram again to go out into the garden! The children were all so good and easy. Perhaps I don't remember the bad times!

It does appear that the physical capacity to achieve tasks in parenting young children – no matter how great they may be – is considered less of a problem by people with multiple sclerosis than the social and psychological aspects of the parenting role. In this respect Cunningham reports a series of problems which the process of parenting presented in her study on a group of people with multiple sclerosis (1977: 66–71). Difficulties arose particularly over discipline. Both mothers and fathers with multiple sclerosis sought to emphasize their role and authority as parents, largely resting on their capacity to discipline and control their children. Disruptive behaviour was seen as occasioned by the parent's disability, rather than by other factors. Inability to confide in parents was similarly explained, with the general view that children were making jaundiced comparisons between their disabled parent and other 'normal' mothers and fathers.

A further problem in relation to older children was the way in which their social roles in the family, and the tasks associated with those roles, might be negotiated and allocated in ways which would perhaps seem inappropriate in other situations. Within the family children could become carers of the parent – in effect parenting the parent – undertaking tasks of a personal and intimate nature which were not socially recognized and legitimized outside the family circle (Cunningham 1977: 67).

In summary Cunningham felt that children and their behaviour were constantly seen through the prism of multiple sclerosis. By implication the parent with the disease appeared to compensate for the weakness of their body by seeking substantially more control over their children's activities than would have otherwise been the case. None the less such parents may feel they need to press the case for their credibility in this situation, not least because of the way that their capacities may be considered by their spouses.

Work and chronic illness: the case of multiple sclerosis

There have been a series of reviews of the employment status of people with the disease. A review of the evidence in 1982 in the USA indicated that in the general population, controlling for age, around 80 per cent of men and 50 per cent of women were employed, while amongst those with the disease the combined figures for men and women ranged, in various studies, from 20 per cent to 30 per cent (LaRocca and Holland 1982: 10). In Davoud and Kettle's study in the United Kingdom in 1980 the figure of employed people with the disease was higher at 40 per cent, although they themselves indicate that the nature of their sample probably seriously underestimated the overall extent of unemployment in this group (1980: 10). In addition both studies suggest that underemployment as well as unemployment is a serious problem, although the former is difficult to assess.

It is easy to assume that there is a direct and unequivocal relationship between level of physical disability and unemployment. However a recent and sophisticated study suggests that only a small proportion of the variation between employed and unemployed people with multiple sclerosis can be explained in this way (LaRocca et al. 1985). They conclude that

only 14 per cent of the variation in employment status of the disabled MS patient can be explained by such disease and demographic factors as disability level, age, education and sex. The patients' premorbid personalities and coping styles, as well as their ability to maintain an image of themselves as productive, working individuals may play a significant role in vocational adaptation.

(LaRocca *et al*. 1985: 210)

Thus they argue that factors in individuals, particularly psychological ones, may have a far greater impact on the likelihood of unemployment than levels of physical disability. While the attribution of a more limited role to the level of physical functioning coincides with many other observations in this book, LaRocca *et al*.'s emphasis on the significance of psychological factors may be overplayed. In brief, they fail to consider the interplay between individual factors, and the broader practices in the employment market which may, in combination, produce the effects which they describe. In this respect Davoud and Kettle's study has the reverse difficulties; it overestimates the degree to which physical capacity itself influences employment status, but does analyse the practices in the employment market – of a formally and informally discriminatory kind – which substantially influence that status. In addition they conclude that many employers are ignorant about the nature and implications of multiple sclerosis, which, with other factors, in itself conditions the kinds of choices that individuals may have available to make – whatever their inclinations (Davoud and Kettle 1980: 9–11).

The kinds of complex negotiations which go on with employers and their difficulties are indicated by Chris:

> I've been moved in my job several times, which is because of the MS, as my employers feel I must be put in a job where it won't matter too much if I should be ill. In a way that's made me lose self-respect and drive, but I appreciate that they are still employing me and I still do good work. . . . I do not feel confident in competing or desiring to compete for another [job], which is probably why I allow myself to be pushed back at work.

Freda found herself in some difficulties in her negotiations when her honesty about her multiple sclerosis had serious consequences she did not anticipate:

> [Multiple sclerosis had been diagnosed when she was medical

secretary to a busy general practice.] I [had] been told to
work less hours – a Catch 22 situation – my doctor [not in the
practice] said, 'Tell them you have MS; they will give you
shorter hours – I would.' I did that and [found] they could not
bend a rule – now they knew I had MS – so if I now went
for a local job (I cannot travel far) they would have to mention
the MS. Who wants to employ someone with MS? I worked
as hard as anyone else and always went on with the exception
of one week off in the years I had MS. I asked my GP for a
job and he said, 'Sorry, not with your medical history'.

Anticipating the kinds of difficulties that Freda had may prompt
people to attempt not to reveal their multiple sclerosis either in
their current job, or when applying for another, as in Georgina's
case:

[after a bad relapse] . . . I started looking for a part-time job.
There was an advertisement in the paper for a person to
'make and measure lung casts'. I replied to the Medical
Research Institute, had an interview, and got the job. I had
put aside my remaining walking stick and felt that there was
no reason to tell my new boss . . . that I had MS. I thought
I would work for a year and then tell him. I did just that. It
made no difference. I am still working there and love it.

The decision about whether to search for a job at all may become
very complex as people try to evaluate their capacities and the
effects that employment may have on their lives. Abby reflects:

I had also planned to combine motherhood and a career – one
reason I had chosen my career was that it offered the
possibility of part-time work in the future – and had imagined
going back to work when the children were settled at school.
I am not at all sure I have the stamina to do both now. Most
mothers face this dilemma but for me there is the added
problem that if I go back to work, then I suffer a relapse, I
really will be condemned to the role of housewife. I would
have a hard time convincing my husband or anyone else that
a job was important to me and that more help on the
domestic front to enable me to continue working would be an
alternative answer.

Whatever the reason for underemployment or unemployment,

the effects on personal and social lives are likely to be profound. Two studies have pointed to the loss of self-image and social role that may occur, particularly for men (Cunningham 1977: 70; I. Robinson, Lawson, and Wynne 1983). Of course it is important to recognize that the effects on the current and potential employment status of those involved in caring for people with multiple sclerosis may be just as great as on those with the disease itself. Raymond indicates how he believes he himself has been diminished through his own work being badly affected:

> My wife's condition began to be such as to demand more and more help and attention and this coincided with the depression in the engineering industry. [He was a managing director of an engineering company in a group.]
>
> Although I obtained the services of two friends to come in two mornings a week each I found that I could not spend long days away from home . . . after several years of loss-making in my company my divisional manager director transferred me to a more routine and mundane job at head office with a drop of salary of 25 per cent.
>
> This was not only a terrible blow to my pride but also affected the economics of running our household. I feel that my wife's illness was used as a matter of convenience simply to reduce the management costs of my company.

Kathy feels bitter about what the disease and her husband in equal measure have done to her own ambitions:

> My main regret in life is never having taken my nursing training . . . if I had my time all over again I would join Queen Alexandra's and travel and get my SRN. . . . I don't want to sound bitter – but I do feel cheated. I can never remember not being married. In this last few years I have become very independent – my husband used to like to keep me under his thumb. Really I suppose if he had not contracted MS we would probably be divorced now . . . my life is now really looking after him – he needs help in nearly every way although he wouldn't admit it for the world. I try to keep cheerful but can't help wondering what life would have been like in the forces, visiting all those places.

Employment can become then a sort of marker for the disease and its effects. The financial consequences of underemployment or unemployment can be very considerable, but it is the effects on self-image and social status which seem particularly critical. The general evidence is that a deterioration in employment status arises from a combination of psychological factors, social constraints, and discrimination in the employment market, rather than directly from changes in physical functioning.

Self and others: the social context and consequences of multiple sclerosis

In this chapter a series of issues have been explored which relate to ways that people with multiple sclerosis, and those with whom they live, work, or come in contact, manage the condition. It has been difficult to separate out the effects of multiple sclerosis from other factors in the kinds of strategies and life-styles that people lead. However, a theme running through the analysis is that, contrary to 'common-sense' views, the level of physical functioning of people with the disease is generally not the decisive factor in itself in decisions or negotiations about those strategies and life-styles. The variation in people's personalities; their attitudes and beliefs; who they marry or who their partners are; their relationships with family, friends, neighbours, and strangers; their social background; and their jobs and relationships with their employers, are likely to have at least as much bearing on life-style as the physical trajectory of the disease.

Chapter five

The experience of managing multiple sclerosis

Explanations and solutions: the quest for the effective management of multiple sclerosis

Solutions to problems, as cures to diseases, are based on some rationale or explanation of the origin of the problem. Such rationales or explanations may precede the finding of a solution, they may follow that solution, or indeed they may indicate in the end why a solution is difficult or impossible to find. The question 'Why me?' is one which is asked with regularity in relation to many life events, not least at the onset of a chronic disease. This personal focus is an essential component of individuals' understanding of their illness.

The question 'Why me?' is one of a sequence of questions asked by people as a preliminary to determining their personal strategy. Helman categorizes these questions as

What has happened?
Why has it happened?
Why has it happened to me?
Why now?
What would happen if nothing were done about it?
What should I do about it?

(Helman 1981: 548)

All of these questions stem from, and relate to, the individual and their situation. The questions are not asked in the abstract. They are filtered through the individual's beliefs, attitudes, and personal experiences.

The cause of multiple sclerosis, for an individual, might be located in a number of explanatory possibilities. At their most general these possibilities can be seen as fourfold (Helman 1984: 75). First, those explanations which are situated in the affected individual or their own actions. Second, those explanations which are situated in the natural world. Third, those explanations which are situated in the social world, where illness is caused by others. Fourth, those explanations which are situated in the supernatural world.

Sally indicated, even through her rational scepticism, that a combination of personal, natural, and social factors might be associated with the genesis of the disease:

> At one point in the time immediately after diagnosis I became convinced that if I had not left Scandinavia – and I hadn't wanted to – I should not have contracted MS. That's patently unreasonable and unfair, as it lays the blame at my husband's door – because he persuaded me to come back to England. I felt this theory was disproved the moment I voiced it, because it sounded ridiculous. The other [idea about the cause of her MS] . . . was that I was being punished for allowing my son to leave and not being a good enough mother.

The initial explanatory framework for others was couched in an apparently rather detached view of the workings of the natural biological environment:

> How do I explain what has happened to me? I certainly don't think it is some visitation by a malevolent God, nor a punishment for sins. I just regard myself as a statistic, absolutely classic, female, middle class, North of England, and there's no reason why I shouldn't get it. How to explain where MS comes from in the first place? This isn't a question which taxes me. I suppose there are just bound to be malfunctions in organic material.

This individual, but somehow externally observed, account is implicitly associated with a low level of personal culpability for the disease. However for many, the causes of their disease, as well as its management, hinge on their 'responsibility' for its onset, even if this responsibility is linked with other factors. Thus Abby suggests:

> I presume, having read pretty widely on the subject recently, that I must have been born with a susceptible genotype; that

I contracted a relevant childhood illness or illnesses (e.g. measles) at an early age; that certain dietary features are not optimal (e.g. insufficient PUFA's [polyunsaturated fatty acids] in the diet – however as a family we ate a lot less animal fat than most and very little fried food as children), and that I chose to lead a very intellectually, emotionally, and physically demanding life-style which was undoubtedly stressful. After leaving school I didn't take regular exercise of any sort other than walking, and although not overweight was not very fit. I can only assume that all these things have a bearing on the development of my MS. The factors that I can change I have tried to change but I am aware that I can't do much about my genes or any virus infections I have had in the past.

A more general formulation of this position is stated by Jim who indicates his commitment to a personal war against the disease, even if he is less precise about the causes of it. He does not feel that 'luck' should be considered as the main factor in the causation of the disease is tenable:

My reaction to having this 'disease' was to do everything in my power to combat it, despite being told frequently not to do so by hospital doctors. I feel sure that the body doesn't just become diseased 'out of the blue' and consequently feel that it can be regenerated and fight off the disease whether it be cancer, arthritis, or MS.

As a generalization it does appear that Jim's view is a very common perspective on both the aetiology and management of multiple sclerosis. This view enables personal sense to be made of a disease for which 'rational' and 'scientific' explanations are not readily available. It also enables the development of a potential feeling of control over some aspects of the situation. The personal costs of 'taking the blame' for the disease in this context seem more than counterbalanced by the possibilities of seizing the initiative in the battle for the future of a declining body.

In the process of developing a way of managing their multiple sclerosis individuals can be argued to be following a similar kind of experimental approach to that engaged in by medical scientists (I. Robinson 1987a). From theories about the cause of their condition they develop hypotheses tested through their actions to derive the most effective strategy for them.

However, this 'lay science' creates particular problems in relationship to medical practice – especially when, as in the case of multiple sclerosis, there are no clear and medically accepted treatment strategies. The combination of a range of scientific theories, and a range of lay theories about the cause of the disease, gives rise to a complex pattern of personal actions and behaviours. In this process the doctor–patient relationship is particularly subject to stress and strain.

Searching for answers: using the medical process

Developing positive doctor–patient relationships in multiple sclerosis depends on what people with the disease want from contact with the medical profession, and whether doctors are able or prepared to give them what they want. The nature of this equation at one level is unequivocal; people want a cure for their disease, and doctors are not able to deliver such a cure. The fact that doctors individually, and medical science in general, cannot at present offer a cure, provides the background against which patients with multiple sclerosis approach their doctors.

In this setting doctors may follow a number of other strategies individually or severally. They may monitor the progress of the disease; they may provide symptomatic relief; they may refer people to other agencies or professions for support; they may offer participation in trials of new drugs or other therapies; or they may offer the consolation and the therapy of understanding and communication itself.

All these options are second best to what many people with the disease really want, and it is not clear whether or to what extent such people can or are prepared to modify their expectations of the doctor in these circumstances. If they do not, Burnfield argues that the doctor can easily become a scapegoat for unrealistic expectations (1985: 62–3). Having 'surrendered oneself to the care of others' in the medical system, as Rosengren puts it (1980: 283), the expected obligations imposed on doctors by those with the disease can be substantial. Only climbing the foothills of symptomatic relief is frustrating to those who wish to climb the mountain of a cure. On the other hand it may be the case that doctors, frustrated by their lack of any real medical control over this chronic progressive condition, minimize, ritualize, and routinize contact with the diagnosed patient. Such contact is maybe unimportant (that is routine) to the doctor but is charged with emotion for the patient. David vividly expresses the poignancy of the patient's role in this continuing round of routine consultations:

> Mentioning doctors raises a whole series of thoughts . . . and there have been a whole series of specialists. . . . All the specialists go through a routine which is now familiar. This involves a wait in a comfortable waiting-room looking at the expensive decor and leafing through copies of *Punch* and *Country Life*. Then there are the now familiar tests involving pins, tuning forks, and rubber hammers to check your reflexes. Then the questions . . .
> 'When was that? And what happened after that episode? . . . I thought you said that happened before? . . . They are difficult to remember accurately.'
> But they also ask more ominous ones like this: 'Can you feel this? . . . Can you hear this? . . . Any trouble with your waterworks? . . . Sex function completely normal is it? . . . Now grip my fingers as hard as you can. . . .'
> Strangely intimate, yet strangely stilted at the same time. But above all saddening and frightening I find. 'Saddening' because I have to live and recall, in some detail, times when I was more carefree and when I could move around far more easily. 'Frightening' because why would he ask about what I can do, unless there's some thought that the answer might have been 'No', or it might be 'No' sometime in the future.

David emphasizes the enormous significance of the ritual of the consultation for the patient. Each time it refocuses attention on the losses that have been sustained; even more worrying, on the losses that may come, and implicitly most concerning of all on the absence of any medical answer to those losses.

People with multiple sclerosis may develop considerable levels of knowledge in relation to their disorder. Geoff indicates how this process works. By utilizing his own experience and undertaking some personal research he had built up a body of knowledge on the drugs he had been given. He had felt sufficiently technically competent to make his own decision confidently on whether to continue taking them:

> Just over two years ago I found the will to come off all the chemical drugs I was taking. I know these things have their

uses but, for me, they complicated my already confused condition. Research had taught me that the corticosteroids are not universally used in the treatment of long-term disease. Many countries have restricted their use except for emergency treatment . . . many experts here and certainly abroad . . . feel this is a wrong usage as the build-up of side-effects can be very detrimental to the patient.

This interest in and pursuit of information on the effects of various therapies is part of the process of personal experimentation mentioned above. It is a process which involves the acquisition of general research knowledge, but knowledge which is filtered and reflected through the prism of deeply personal concern about the individual's own future. The research quest is therefore important, committed, directed, and specific.

Such a personal research strategy is also used by others as a means of adjudicating between the benefits and costs of medically proffered therapies. Medical interventions to produce symptomatic relief, amongst which might be included drug therapies to ameliorate attacks of multiple sclerosis, are areas of medical care which many people with the disease have experienced. Of particular importance here is the medical administration of steroids, which have often been given in an attempt to reduce the severity and length of attacks of the disease. This is one of the very few therapies found to be effective in this respect in clinical trials. As Geoff reports above there may be potentially disturbing side-effects of steroids, although with corresponding short-term benefits for some people. It is clear that the balance between costs and benefits is carefully weighed up, with decisions about continuing with the course of treatment apparently as much in the patient's as the doctor's hands. Annette illustrates a thoughtful approach to the use of a steroid (ACTH):

[After being seriously disabled by an attack of MS] a course of ACTH was given. This, after feeling quite ill for the first two to three weeks due to the side-effects, gave me a boost. . . . As the course of ACTH progressed I gained more and more energy and felt quite perky, but had to have rests during the day . . . my disability has worsened and the ACTH [has been] used more frequently, but not with such marked results as when I first had it. . . . I do not feel inclined to have further ACTH as I feel I have had too much over the past few years, even though it gives me a booster feeling and improves my mobility, by enabling me to stand more easily.

Others have tried ACTH and found that the side-effects for them outweigh the possible advantages. Thus Nigel says:

The steroids for me were a bit of a disaster. As well as the usual acne and digestive problems, they affected me psychiatrically which I was quite unprepared for, and I vowed never to take them again.

On the other hand there are those who have a much more positive attitude towards ACTH such as Lesley:

I got MS in 1976 although it was not diagnosed then. . . . I had a course of ACTH and got almost completely better.

The conclusion that might be drawn from these accounts is that each person places the use of the drug in the context of his or her own expectations, life experiences, and those aspects of health that he or she values most. Most people, in common with medical scientists, may have difficulty at any one time in distinguishing the effects of drugs (or other therapies) on themselves from naturally occurring remissions in the disease, or from other simultaneous but unrelated events. However it would be wrong to conclude that this distinction is not possible for individuals over a period of time, in the careful pattern of experimentation that many people pursue.

The problem of people not doing precisely what their doctors advise (or direct) – as indicated in the actions of some of those quoted above – is normally considered to be a problem of 'non-compliance' amongst those formally concerned with health care. This view implies that the only legitimate and the pre-eminent objective of the doctor--patient relationship is that which is determined by the expertise of the doctor. In general, and particularly in the case of chronic illness, there are substantial grounds for arguing for the mutual legitimacy of both patients' and doctors' agendas and objectives, and for a mutuality of expertise in the accomplishment of a difficult task. The indications are in chronic illness that often both doctors and patients have individually inadequate resources to accomplish the goals in the clinical setting that they each seek. The pooling of their respective and complementary expertise may facilitate the achievement of some of those goals.

Interpersonal aspects of medical care

None the less it appears to be the interpersonal skill of the doctor on which a great premium is placed – in particular the doctor's frankness, caring concern for the individual, and preparedness to engage in a mutual interchange of information (I. Robinson 1986). The perceived absence of some of these wished-for features may fracture doctor–patient relationships, and may affect the doctor's capacity to work in a technically competent way, as in Elsie's case:

> if only the doctors could talk to me, explain more. People I spoke to had heard of the illness but it was a closed subject, like the time I thought I had a chill. I kept passing water and wetting myself, so I got some barley and nursed a hot-water bottle for three days. Then I went to my GP who said, 'What do you expect? It's to do with your complaint'. What do you expect I thought at home? I don't know what to expect – no one tells me anything. How am I expected to know? My anger seemed to mentally give me strength – I'd show them, I won't give in – me in a wheelchair – never.

That moral support is needed from doctors to help continually with the struggle with the disease is emphasized in the comments of Lisa and Zoe. Lisa has been fortunate to have a relationship with her consultant in which the communication is very positive:

> I wrote a long letter to Dr X today, requesting an appointment with him . . . there is no need to see him often. I just feel a need to speak to him. More than anyone else in my life I get such a tremendous satisfaction from just speaking to him. I don't know why. Probably because I think he genuinely cares what happens to me.

Zoe on the other hand feels

> Everything I know and have found out about MS I have had to research for myself. I have never had a doctor who has sat down at any time with me and talked about my hopes and fears and how I feel. I think this is very bad. Fortunately I

have had my husband for comfort, but for anyone on their own it must be a terrible thing to live with. . . . Doctors I have come across seem to say, 'Well, you have MS, go home and live with it'.

The problems of communication perceived by patients with multiple sclerosis in doctor–patient relationships seem not surprisingly to be generally acute and difficult and do not relate only to the time of diagnosis. In the case of multiple sclerosis the curative thrust of much modern medicine passes the patient by, while at the same time the major specialist medical skills are hospital based – the home of curative medicine. To the extent that the medical and perhaps especially the neurological emphasis can be redirected from diagnosis towards rehabilitation, and from cure towards care, the problems of communication between doctors and patients may be improved. However there is a paradox here, for the idea of a cure is as important to many patients as it is to those professionally involved in modern medicine. Thus the mutual expectations of both parties to the medical consultation may ensure that the transition to a different form of relationship is difficult and painful.

In this situation many patients seek alternative avenues of support for their objectives to those provided by doctors and the medical system.

Using alternatives: rational eclecticism in personally managing multiple sclerosis

Most health care, whether in relation to multiple sclerosis or any other condition, takes place outside the domain of scientific medicine. The iceberg of contact with the formal medical system has already been referred to in Chapter 2. As McEwen, Martini, and Wilkins indicate: 'it appears that most families deal almost continually with symptoms and illness'. They also state that 'Self-care is the true first level of health care and comprises numerically the major portion of the system. There are many more people caring for their own complaints than there are attending health professionals' (1983: 56).

Against this background of a considerable and continuing degree of self-assessment, self-diagnosis, and self-care in all kinds of ill health, the exploration and use of 'alternative' therapies by those with multiple sclerosis is unsurprising – at least to people with the disease. It appears that people engage in self-medication both in relation to medically trivial symptoms, and in relation to medically serious – especially chronic – conditions. Of the six reasons identified by McEwen, Martini, and Wilkins for self-medication (1983: 70–1) at least four might appositely apply to many of those with multiple sclerosis; these are first, concerns that the doctor's time might be being wasted; second, expectations that nothing can really be done; third, poor experience with previous medical contacts; and fourth, problems of inconvenient access to doctors compared to alternative possibilities.

In the broadest sense self-care in relation to multiple sclerosis can be taken to include those strategies undertaken through the choice and actions of individuals outside the framework of conventional medical advice or recommendation. Extrapolating from research into people's general health-related behaviour, it might be expected that some of these 'alternative' strategies would be used simultaneously with the recommendations of doctors and other strategies used in place of those recommendations, or in the absence of them (Anderson *et al.* 1977). People's exploration of alternative approaches to their multiple sclerosis might be prompted by their bad experiences with what conventional medicine had to offer, as in Kim's situation:

[After a bad attack of MS which meant five months in the hospital where she was diagnosed] . . . I was given every tranquillizer they could think of and ACTH but when nothing helped I was packed off to a rehabilitation centre full of people with MS, stroke, and the like. It was a most depressing place and a poster on the wall said, 'Smile and be happy – things might be worse'. So I smiled and *was* happy, and behold things did get worse! This attitude made me so mad that I determined to get out . . . and when the shock started to wear off I began vaguely to wonder what *I could do*.

Everyone kept saying, 'Come to terms' or 'Accept it' and seemed to mean to sit back and do nothing . . . we read an article in the *Sunday Times* . . . and sent away for information . . . we got hold of Judy Graham's book [*Multiple Sclerosis – A Self-Help Guide to its Management*] . . . this explained the rationale for a low animal fat diet and supplementation with gamma-linoleic acid. I now began to have real hope and the black bouts of despair lessened. . . . I realized it would take a long time to show benefit, but I had no choice but to keep plodding on.

Then I saw an advertisement in our local newspaper for interested people to start a nutrition and exercise group. I joined and we soldier on together and still do. Much easier in company. At the same time a friend of mine who had taken a course [in yoga for MS] started a . . . class in yoga for the disabled. We all find that helpful too. The philosophy perhaps more than the postures. I began slowly to improve.

Then the HBO [hyperbaric oxygen] therapy came up, which after the Dundee study [a small-scale trial of HBO] became a viable proposition. . . . I began to feel at last I was getting somewhere and had something to offer. . . . I feel full of hope for the future.

It is not clear to what extent Kim has radically improved her physical condition, but in some ways this is only one component of the change that she feels had been wrought. The transformation of her views about her situation and her future seem largely to do with her active involvement in the management of her own life, the sense of personal control this gives her, and the legitimizing and endorsement of her views by like-minded others.

In Kerrie's comments below it can be seen that she is using both prescribed medication and a whole series of other therapies. She is continually experimenting to get what she considers to be the best mix of strategies for a range of symptoms.

[Even though I was on daily injections of ACTH] twenty-one months ago I started HBO treatment and after the initial month I have been going once a week for top-ups. . . . After about a year I realized my bladder function was better and that each week I was getting a slight lift which diminished the following week. There is a slight but noticeable improvement before and after each session that is noticeable to others as well as myself.

On the principle that every little helps I had a cytoxic blood test done a year ago. It was found I was sensitive to [a range of foods] . . . so these were out, and an unpleasant feeling I had when I woke at night at the top of my throat and at the left side of my tongue, and a sniffly nose, vanished almost immediately. Before then my bowels would move every three or four – even five or six – days but have over the year improved to virtually daily. For four or five years I and the whole family have been eating a Judy Graham type diet . . . and the general health of the family is good. . . .

With the colder weather in mid-October I found that there was a slight but almost daily improvement in walking and wanting to do things, so much so that after a month I stopped the daily ACTH injections. Then I found I had trouble getting down the stairs, as well as the normal trouble going up – it was as if I ran out of energy on the way down. When the injections were resumed I got further and further downstairs, then into the kitchen, and after a time had no trouble at all. In a way it was useful, that experience, to discover the injections do seem to be really necessary for me. The slight but more or less continuous improvement has continued.

This kind of experimental approach appears to be a very common strategy in the personal management of multiple sclerosis. It leads to an eclecticism in which formal information and advice from a doctor – whether general physician or specialist – is only one amongst many sources of information. In the search for a combination of strategies which together are associated with improvements – or at least no significant worsening of the condition, itself deemed an improvement over what might have been – there is a constant ebb and flow of interest in new possibilities from any source, or old possibilities which might be reworked into a new combination of therapies. Plateaux in the progression of the disease, or gentle (and generally temporary) gradients of improvement, may be associated with a more stable set of personal strategies, although these are likely to be re-evaluated at the first sign of any change. Indeed such a flexibility in approach seems considered worth pursuing almost at any cost. Against the probability of inevitable decline, present or future, and the negligible immediate possibility of finding a cure, the more substantial possibility of finding some means of checking symptoms associated with the progression of the disease, is still an objective of substance for the individual. In any case the personal benefits of re-establishing a sense of control over life are considerable. Moreover even if no benefit of either sort were to accrue from operating this kind of strategy, to have undertaken it cannot in retrospect be gainsaid, as Alan succinctly indicates:

> Find out your favourite alternative medicine and pursue it with all you've got. Acupuncture, reflexology, homeopathy, whatever is your taste, try it; it may not work, but it will do no harm and make you feel better.

Doctors and others professionally concerned with the management of those with multiple sclerosis often find these common kinds of personal approaches to dealing with the disease hard to understand. Burnfield, a doctor but also someone who has multiple sclerosis, bases his grave concern about what he takes to be people's 'irrational' use of medically dubious strategies on the idea that

> Most people have little concept of what scientific proof is all about. They are more likely to decide whether or not a particular treatment is effective from the anecdotes and stories heard from their friends and acquaintances, however bizarre the story may be.
>
> (Burnfield 1985: 44)

Burnfield goes on to argue for the rigorous scientific testing of new therapies, and for people with multiple sclerosis to make their choice of therapies solely on the basis of their formal scientific validity (1985: 44–7). This is a position that is entirely tenable within the logic of scientific medicine, and would probably be held by the vast majority of those doctors working in clinical practice and medical research. However it is not necessarily incompatible with the explanation and understanding of the actions of the many people who do seek out and use what may be described medically as dubious therapies.

First, as has been argued above, many people – perhaps most people – have always employed a variety of approaches to their symptoms and illness, only a minority of which involve doctors or the formal medical system. Therefore if people with multiple sclerosis continue to use a multiplicity of means to manage their situation they are not doing something new, aberrant, or extraordinary, for they are likely to be following health practices established before they acquired the disease. Those strategies may be different in degree, or be more socially visible, but they are not different in kind from those previous practices. Indeed statistically it is likely to be more aberrant to pursue only strategies advised by doctors.

Second, although medical science may have established a formal and laudable structure for testing the efficacy of new therapies for multiple sclerosis, people with the disease have to rely at present on the promise rather than the achievements of scientific medicine. In this situation people may argue that even though they believe in the principle of scientific research, and are anxious, for example, to participate in clinical trials, they are faced with present problems and bleak futures which warrant – perhaps necessitate – their experimentation with unconventional and untried therapies.

Third, and following from the second point, the agenda and objectives of people with the disease may be different from those generally held by doctors and medical scientists. Although as was indicated above the objective of a cure is never far from the minds of people with the disease, their doctors, and medical scientists, those having multiple sclerosis may have a set of other objectives (Zola 1973). Such objectives may be associated particularly with managing the disease in the context of their overall lives. The goal might be to gain a sense of control over events, to be continually and actively involved in health maintenance, to show others and themselves that they have not 'given in', or to gain the support and succour of like-minded people in this process. These objectives may be moulded round symptom control but none the less form a significantly separate agenda.

The ways in which many people with multiple sclerosis use 'alternative' therapies is of great concern to many doctors, as has been indicated. Such concern is expressed, amongst other things, as anxiety about the efficacy of the therapies, the cost of them for patients, and the dangers that patients may face in their use. These views are based in part on the medical ignorance imputed to patients and their susceptibility to extra-medical claims. Although susceptibility to such pressures at times of stress and despair is indeed possible, the view that all or many people with multiple sclerosis who engage in 'alternative' medicine are ignorantly gullible can be sustained only by a very narrow, partisan, and arguably incorrect reading of the nature, role, and place of scientific medicine. The contentious debate at heart may be more about the control of the territorial boundaries of multiple sclerosis, over which neither doctors, medical scientists, nor patients can establish effective practical supremacy.

Life-style changes: diet and exercise

In the complex landscape of managerial strategies used in relation to multiple sclerosis, those related to nutrition and exercise might be thought to bridge the boundary between 'alternative' and conventional medicine. Such strategies both reflect features peculiar to the disease itself – in particular both scientific and personal ideas about its genesis, and more general concerns about healthy living and healthy life-styles.

Food, as Helman points out, is not a simple substance. In addition to being a basic source of nutrition it carries with it symbolic meanings, and just as important is located in and reinforces social organization and practices (Helman 1984: 23). Mobility, movement, and exercise are similarly symbolically and socially important, and carry with them, and reinforce values about social roles. None the less both food and exercise can be seen as elements of the natural world, neither 'alternative' nor conventional in their basic connotations.

The onset of multiple sclerosis is treated by some as a failure in these 'natural' elements either caused fortuitously and by chance or caused partly by their own actions. This possible fusion of personal responsibility and natural imbalances is a powerful incentive to modify attitudes and behaviour in relation to diet and exercise. Such a change may be reinforced by several factors such as the dissemination of the results of recent scientific research on the causes and treatment of the multiple sclerosis (Matthews *et al*. 1985: 250–5); the development of a generally sympathetic 'self-care' ideology; the availability and endorsement of particular diets by some people with the disease, and by the more general consciousness of the relationship between diet and exercise and health. As impaired mobility is one of the most common and visible features of the disease there is a special incentive to pursue strategies, perhaps involving particular forms of exercise, which might remedy or contain this problem.

The modification of pre-existing patterns of belief and behaviour in relation to diet and exercise is often not easy. Dee's account reveals an array of difficulties, both for her personally and for those around her which ensued when she made dramatic changes in her life-style:

> My reaction to the diagnosis was striking. Everyone around me, family and friends, wanted me to take things easily almost as though I should resign myself to it, and, for three months, I did.
>
> Then once I started back at work my attitude altered. If I was going to be a cripple I was going to enjoy myself until that happened. For the first time in my life I began to do very exhausting sport. I took up weightlifting training four or five times a week, and I pushed myself to the limit. I stuck obsessively to a new low-fat MS diet to the degree that I now have a 'hang-up' over food and am currently having psychotherapy in this connection. I had never played any sport before except at school. People thought I was mad, but I began to feel so much better, and life took on a new meaning. My theory was that if the body was in the best possible condition, I would have more chance of 'surviving' another attack when it came. The family were all against this at first. I think they felt I was going against the rules, and [I] would bring on another attack myself, but as I improved they accepted it. . . .
>
> Looking back, it's difficult to say how I feel. I certainly think that the diet and exercise programme improved my general health and perhaps this in itself 'prevented' any further attacks.

The interlocking nature of managerial strategies is clearly indicated in Dee's account. Not only are there multiple strategies employed, but also they are to a large degree contingent on each other. Indeed in Dee's circumstances the exercise programme and the diet were both necessary means to her specific objective of ensuring that her body was 'in the best possible condition' to resist future attacks of the disease. This particular philosophy appears to be employed as a firm and secure bedrock strategy, against which other more esoteric, marginal, or contentious managerial approaches might be circumspectly used. In other words such a basic strategy may allow people to experiment more, secure in the knowledge that they are sensibly accomplishing basic body maintenance. The possible benefits of other strategies are therefore bonuses, or, to use an inapposite metaphor, are the icing on the cake.

Dee's approach also has the virtue of apparently reasserting personal control over the natural forces which are out of control in the disease itself, a point specifically taken up by Jim:

> At present I follow a strict therapy – the Gerson therapy – which was first used in cancer. Having something to work at is a tremendous boost and I am totally convinced that it helps me to maintain a very positive outlook. I have discovered self-discipline which I never knew I had and in fact my life and life-style have changed radically over the past two and a half years.

Dee's account above further emphasizes the social context of her actions. She indicates that she refused to accept the way that her family and friends defined her role, and stridently went 'against the rules' to force a change in that definition, at some risk it appears to herself. However she self-evidently considers the risk from attempting to change others' perceptions lower than the risk of remaining the prisoner of the existing perceptions. For Ilsa a social interaction with her consultant precipitated her dietary strategy, contrary, it appears, to his intentions:

> I had a return visit to my miserable neurologist. 'Is diet any good?' 'Well,' he said, 'Some people think it has good effects, but who wants to have Flora on their peas instead of butter?' 'I do,' I almost shouted, 'If it will keep me from a wheelchair.' So I started on the Roger McDougall gluten-free, fat-free, sugar-free diet, with his vitamin supplements. I've been on it ever since. No cheating . . . never. . . . I stick to my diet. If it hasn't done any good, it hasn't done any harm.

Dietary strategies in the management of multiple sclerosis are commonly associated with broader personal philosophies of life, as a number of the accounts quoted above indicate. There are few accounts which indicate that supervision or advice has been given on these matters by those professionally concerned with matters of diet – for example nutritionists in hospitals. This is likely to be because the specific dietary management of multiple sclerosis has not been accepted in the majority of hospitals as a legitimate and separate task. The main mechanism of advice and support has been through published diets written largely as a result of personal experience with the disease, or more recently through the specific espousal of and organizational support for the dietary management of multiple sclerosis by a British voluntary organization, ARMS (Action for Research into Multiple Sclerosis).

The problems of bodily decline in multiple sclerosis are as much to be seen in problems of muscular control and function, as in any other parts of the body. Such decline is particularly hard for people to manage, for it may often occur in the prime of life, and therefore be 'unnatural' (see Chapter 3). The attempt to restore 'natural' muscular control and function is a prime aim of many people with the disease – as in Dee's case above. Although such problems may be tackled indirectly through diet, other personal strategies rely heavily, and sometimes exclusively, on a direct approach to the difficulties.

In conventional medicine the main professional avenue through which remedial help might be obtained for problems of defective muscular movement and mobility is physiotherapy. In an Australian study on the perceptions of people with multiple sclerosis about the use of physiotherapy Simons comments on a series of issues (1984c). He indicates that most people started physiotherapy with high expectations of improvement, some of which were fulfilled; others wished physiotherapy had been obtained earlier with the feeling that improvement might have been even greater; others found that physiotherapy introduced physical demands on them which they felt worsened their condition, at least temporarily; while yet others, particularly the more severely affected, felt that physiotherapists viewed them as lost causes and did not give them the help they needed.

It is difficult to extrapolate directly from one study; none the less the broad findings are reflected in the comments and observations of the autobiographies and other data used in this study. Physiotherapy is a practice which is largely based in the curative rather than rehabilitative (or alleviative) paradigms of scientific medicine (Alaszewski 1979). In this position it is more difficult for many physiotherapists to accept a continuing role in a progressive condition like multiple sclerosis, where the work in the longer term is almost entirely alleviative. It is not surprising therefore to find people with multiple sclerosis who feel that their needs are not being met by physiotherapists, or that demands are being made of them which do not accord with their wishes. It is also the case that physiotherapy is a labour-intensive medical practice, with that labour in the public medical system in short supply. Thus a combination of shortage of resources and a generally different view of their role may mean that it is the exception rather than the rule that people with the disease find their expectations satisfied. There are satisfied people such as Rachel, however, who appreciate the caring involved as much as the technical skills available:

> The physios are a tremendous help to me. Always so kind, patient and practical. I see them once a month for a check up. I really don't know what I would do without them.

In a quest to get beyond the technical skills associated with physiotherapy – which in any case may be in short supply and of an inappropriate kind – to something in which a personal philosophy of life can be incorporated together with exercise, and something which encourages personal rather than professional control, many people with multiple sclerosis have turned to yoga. A subculture of people has developed who have a special affinity for this mode of managing their multiple sclerosis. This account by Veronica expresses, in slightly more philosophical terms than most, the virtues of yoga for her:

> In the summer of 1981 I had my first stay in the Yoga Community . . . who take a special interest in MS. . . . I planned to use my stays as a real attempt 'to be' to balance all the 'doing' for the rest of the year: I needed to see that what I am matters more than what I do. [I like] the simplicity and peace of the community. . . . The balance and harmony of the yoga way of life is very appealing and something I try to incorporate into my daily life at home each day, aiming to balance 'being' and 'doing' each day and making enjoyment as important an aim as 'working'. My spiritual life is the all-important an aim as 'working'. My spiritual life is the all-important force which motivates the rest of my life. The physical side of yoga has a natural appeal for the feeling of well-being that it engenders, which is a very good alternative for me to ballet. . . . I was pleased to find I could substitute yoga postures each day at home for the more demanding ballet exercises I couldn't do any more.

There are a range of reasons why yoga appears to be particularly attractive to people with multiple sclerosis. As Veronica indicates, yoga seems to emphasize 'being' rather than 'doing', a philosophy which coincides with the increasingly restricted capacities of people with the disease to 'do'; it may be adapted easily to the particular physical capacities of the individual, no matter how restricted they may be; it emphasizes the capacity to synthesize the mind and body to overcome those factors unbalancing or afflicting the body; it also appears to emphasize the virtues of separation from the everyday world in meditation or yoga exercises – a separation which many in ordinary life might otherwise experience as a vice into which they were forced by the effects of their condition, or the prejudices of others. Other perceived virtues may relate to the ability of yoga to provide a rationale both for the genesis of the disease, and a change in life-style which would in any case have to be accomplished; its 'naturalness'; and the eclectic way it can either be used as a philosophy of life, or as a limited but effective source of exercises.

Given this apparently formidable list of attractions of yoga for people with multiple sclerosis – particularly in the absence of a medically validated cure – it is perhaps understandable why the use and value of yoga should be so widely reported, compared to the evaluation of physiotherapy. It seems to offer an alternative framework within which the real bodily decline experienced with the disease can be managed within the context of the individual's own resources, although few people may use yoga in such an all-embracing way.

Management of mind and body

Managing multiple sclerosis involves consideration of many different but closely related aspects of life. It also implies coming to terms with the containment of the disease rather than finding its cure, and living with a continuing process rather than with a speedy resolution of difficulties.

The process of containment involves managing the personal meaning of the disease – understanding where it has come from, what it means now, and what it will mean in the future. It involves managing social relationships and the social consequences of the disease. It involves managing practical day-to-day activities. It involves managing symptoms and consequences of the disease. It most of all involves managing the absence of a medically recognized cure.

This process involves continual thought in which a crucial feature is how personal control can best be established. Such control is often seen as residing in a secure and solid mental approach to the disease which depends in the end on the internal resources of the person concerned, however supportive other managerial strategies might be. In these circumstances there is a belief that the right mental attitude is crucial. For example Pauline has worked hard to establish a plausible strategy which works for her:

> I tried looking to God for help but got none and now I think the answer is in me. I have overcome plenty of disasters and can manage this one, but only if my 'mind power works' and I don't deteriorate any more. . . . I cannot explain what has happened to me, just describing it has been difficult enough, although I think about it often enough. I like positive statements such as 'When the going gets tough, the tough get going' and 'Surprise yourself each day with your own courage'. I think there is a certain arrogance in me that I have the need to do everything well, including looking good, having a lovely home . . . playing the piano well. . . . In my black times this is a problem, looking good when you seldom go out, playing the piano to no one, having unexpressed views on everything, but I still go on doing it. . . . I have come to the conclusion I am doing it all for myself. . . . I think my positive attitude is geared up to not letting my illness develop in certain ways rather than coping with them should they happen. I have visited some local sufferers in a very bad condition, and thinking 'I won't be as ill as that' is my way of coping. I know I couldn't cope with not being able to read at all, not being able to see television at all, peeing all over the place, etc. I will just have to make sure I stay as I am – bad enough though that is, I can cope.

Pauline indicates that her strategy is not as secure as she would wish. It is constantly under assault from the attrition of her body. Indeed she has set up the equation between her mind and body in such a way as to perpetually run the risk of having it undermined. If her body deteriorates, as she puts it, her 'mind power' hasn't worked. However, she has allowed herself what might be seen as a second line of defence in setting her own condition in the framework of other 'sufferers' who were worse than her.

The strategy of mental control of the disease can be threatened in some unexpected ways, as Beth indicates:

> Now however all this hope [of compensating for the body with the mind] has been frighteningly undermined with a new development. My mind is now affected and is at present deteriorating slowly but steadily. It's not much, I think, but enough. Yes, I can write all this, I can even do the *Times* crossword sometimes, but I find difficulty calculating my change and forgetting things. I forget what we are having for supper in the middle of preparing it, I forget what I am doing, even stop in mid-sentence and forget what I'm saying. I'm fine early in the day but as the day goes on and fatigue sets in it gets more difficult.

This change that Beth has documented would be the most threatening of all to many people with multiple sclerosis, for it hits hard at the one feature of people's lives which appears to transcend the actual or imminent decline of the body. None the less there is some formal evidence that cognitive abilities, and particularly memory, are affected in a proportion of people with the disease (Grant 1986). Losing cognitive capacities may not lead to such a dramatic self-evaluation as Beth has undergone but it suggests that the fortress of the mind is not as easily defensible from the ravages of the disease as people may wish.

Following on from these comments David muses briefly but poignantly on the relationship of the mind to the body, and summarizes the dilemma:

> there is the perfectly sensible assertion from almost everyone that the mind and the body are linked. I think that's true. But if a healthy body means a healthy mind, then what does it mean if you have an unhealthy body?

In conclusion people with multiple sclerosis may adopt a multiplicity of strategies for the personal management of the disease. Many of these lie outside the relatively narrow confines of conventional scientific medicine. Part of the reason why the search for strategies extends out beyond the conventional medical system not only lies in the absence of a cure and hard-pressed resources within that environment, but also is because the objectives and aims of people with the disease seem so different from those of many of the professionals engaged formally with the condition. In particular the link between the body and mind, so crucial to people with multiple sclerosis, seems to be denied or minimized in that formal professional environment. In this situation it is the sources of support that people with the disease turn to that are now considered.

Chapter six

Sources of support: possibilities and problems

Expectations and experience of support from medical services

Despite major difficulties often experienced in the relationship between doctors and some people with multiple sclerosis evident from the preceding discussion, the importance of this relationship as a potential source of support needs to be recognized. In Elian and Dean's survey (1983), doctors – both general practitioners and consultants – appeared as the most frequent professional contacts amongst all professional groups, for people with the disease. More recent research has suggested that general practitioners in particular have a particularly high level of contact of people with multiple sclerosis (Radford and Trew 1987: 44–5). As the focal point of access to many health-related services, and to possible means of symptomatic relief, such contact should be seen as unsurprising despite the concerns about the communicative competence of doctors expressed by people with multiple sclerosis in Chapters 2 and 5. However, the relatively high rate of contact, in the context of concern about its rewards by some people with the disease, indicates an area of ambiguity which deserves further exploration.

The basis of the bargain of support between the patient and the doctor is a complex one. At one level it may be centred on the exchange of the fruits of medical skill and expertise, for the surrender of the patient's personal responsibility. It is not clear how many people with multiple sclerosis do surrender this responsibility and gain this type of support – partly on the basis that the fruits of medical expertise are currently small and often unappetizing for those with the disease. However, this view of a relatively crude bargain of support engineered through the doctor–

patient relationship almost certainly underestimates the more subtle – and supportive – aspects of the relationship.

A common pattern has been for neurologists to diagnose the disease, and general practitioners to alleviate or manage the symptoms as presented to them by people with the disease. This separation of diagnosis from management, generally undertaken by separate doctors in different settings, allows people with multiple sclerosis to make different judgements about them. In these different kinds of judgements it is the general practitioner who is generally perceived as the more supportive – perhaps understandably in view of the findings of Elian and Dean who say, in commenting on what seemed (to them) a relatively high degree of contact by people with their consultants after their diagnosis:

> Since little can be done for a multiple sclerosis patient by a consultant once he has confirmed the diagnosis, it seems that most of these patients were seeing their consultants too often. A majority thought the visits were a formality only.
>
> (Elian and Dean 1983: 1,092)

It is quite possible these patients were right in their judgement about the visits being a formality. The consultant neurologist, apart from being in an organizationally more distant position from a patient, is largely (perhaps only) involved with the diagnostic process, in which social rather than medical contact with the person with the disease may be limited in duration and substance. However, decisions may be taken about the release of information on the diagnosis, which above all hinge on social and personal judgements about individuals and their families. The available information on which to make these judgements can be limited and, from the evidence in Chapter 3, mismanaged. In these circumstances the contrast between the virtues of general practitioners and vices of hospital consultants can be cemented, as in Janice's case:

> The main reason I would like to have been told by my GP is that I know and respect him, and he in turn treats me as a responsible, intelligent person, spending time to explain things to me clearly. The worst part about finding out through my husband being told first was that it seemed to cast me as a fool who could not take it, and I certainly felt like an outsider when I realized what had been done. I have still not seen the

neurologist since he told my husband and that seems an added insult – as though once he has made his diagnosis and 'chickened out' of telling me himself I am of no medical interest to him at all, and my care can be tossed over to an assistant.

If the implications of recent research could be incorporated into practice (e.g. Poser *et al.* 1983; Elian and Dean 1985; I. Robinson 1986; Radford and Trew 1987), such situations might be made less common than they appear to be at present. People with the disease themselves generally have a clear and relatively uniform view of what is required to feel they have received greater support from their consultant (I. Robinson 1986). The comments of several other people emphasize the keys, for them, to a good relationship with a consultant at this difficult time. Jay suggests that the consultant should

Answer the patient's questions honestly. That was not my own experience. . . . Follow-up consultatations should be arranged so that questions can be asked once the initial shock has worn off (this is for people who are 'shocked' rather than 'relieved'). The latter might be more able to ask sensible questions and take in the answers. Information about the MS Society and ARMS might be a good idea. I feel one should be told that there are 'unorthodox' treatments and pointed in the direction of the information if they wish to follow it up. After all the 'establishment' medical profession has little to offer.

Andy comments that the consultant ought to

Explain the illness in full because I am sure that most people want to know. To give the person time initially to take it all in, because having to cope with MS is such a shock. To be given a feeling of hope because even with the strongest will power it is so easy to feel so lost at times. To be made to feel that they are no less a person for having MS.

Debbie felt that her consultant nearly got it right for her, although she would have liked further explanation about the disease:

My doctor was very good in that he invited me to go and see him whenever I had doubts or questions. He did not explain too well about the meaning of the disease. I would have liked

to have been recommended some reading material relevant
to the disease. This is only because I am not very good at
taking a lot of new facts into my mind verbally. I prefer to
be able to repeatedly dip into a book and look up information.

Linda echoes this point, but also links it to the need to offer
encouragement:

It would help tremendously if the doctor suggested that the
patient should learn as much as possible about the MS so
that they were not afraid of it through ignorance, instead of
so many doctors who say, 'You must learn to live with it –
there is no cure at present', and not give any help or
encouragement in coping with the problems as they arise.

And Meg raises an important and often underrated issue in her
point about the personal reactions of the consultant to the stress
of the occasion when the diagnosis is given:

they should try and hide any embarrassment they feel which
could prevent you from 'letting go'.

In general practice, as in a hospital setting, it becomes clear to
people with multiple sclerosis when doctors are being helpful and
supportive and when they are not. Diverse views about the role
of general practitioners may be expressed. Bobby has found a
particularly helpful medical confidante and supporter:

I was discharged from X hospital and within three years had
three further attacks. I consulted my GP on each occasion
and on the second occasion we discussed my condition . . . he
explained the probable cause and effect and advised me to
avoid stress, tension, and overtiredness. In the discussion it
came out that there was no known cure. He was very
concerned, as he is now, that he could not give me more
positive advice or help in the management of this disease.

Since that date my wife and I (without whom I could not
have coped) have obtained and read many articles on this
disease. We have tried, in conjunction with my GP, many
ways to cope with the disease, medication, diets, vitamin and
mineral supplements, in an effort to retard the progress of the
complaint. My GP is fully aware that I am willing to try
anything and is very willing to assist in anything new that
appears on the scene.

On the other hand there are those such as Rita who fail to find either the communicative – or perhaps even the technical – support they feel is due to them from their general practitioners:

> at work I couldn't see; on contacting my doctor I was told 'Oh it's the MS'. I thought that I had cystitis; I was told 'Oh it's the MS, I will give you some tablets'. I drop things and have severe pains in my arms: 'Oh it's the MS'. I feel there is no point in seeing my doctor about anything because 'It's the MS'. Because apart from dragging legs and weak arms and legs there is nothing to show – doctors need to cure people and you must just get on with it.

Carrie puts the point succinctly:

> My GP blithely says that he knows very little about MS – with the inference that he cares even less.

In this situation people just 'get on with it', as Rita puts it. They use other resources that may be available, especially including their own capacities, to ensure that their lives are lived as well as they possibly can be.

Doing it yourself – the organization of everyday life

The practical organization of everyday life for people with multiple sclerosis is largely undertaken outside the context of medical care and requires special, sometimes spectacular, attention to ensure a successful and orderly personal world. For some this adjustment to disability and its consequences is occasional and slight; for others it is regular and major. The adjustment may be predictable and attainable. For others it may be unpredictable and in effect unattainable. It may be capable of being achieved alone, with the informal help of others, or require the intervention of an outside agency, or through a consummation of all three. Thus the practical as well as the emotional adjustments required in organizing a life with multiple sclerosis are multiple, complex, and contingent on each other.

Sources of support in this situation are also likely to be multiple, complex, and contingent. These sources of support may only be brought into play when problems can be isolated and identified and when solutions, or at least means towards solutions, can be found. The role of outside agencies in this process is a distinctly problematic matter. Blaxter found fifty-nine different agencies in the city where her research was undertaken, all of whose functions, at least in part, were to help with problems caused by sickness or disability (1976: 18). It is likely that a similar situation obtains elsewhere. This system of agencies has materialized with different objectives, at different historical points, for different client groups, with different procedures, and with different structures. It requires therefore a feat of some magnitude to be able to draw efficiently on the appropriate sets of health and social services for particular personal needs.

In this context it is not surprising that Elian and Dean's study found a generally confused picture of support for people with multiple sclerosis, with clear inadequacies of provision overall; as much due to misunderstandings, incompetence, and organizational problems, as to do with the level of resources (1983). Radford and Trew's study (1987) echoes many of these findings. In many respects the complex range of problems of people with multiple sclerosis have constituted, it can be argued, a particularly difficult test for outside agencies (Kraft, Freal, and Coryell 1986). None the less the extent to which people with the disease constantly 'rediscover' solutions to similar problems suggests that the statutory and voluntary agencies concerned are failing to meet a considerable level of unmet need for practical support. This was evident in Elian and Dean's study, for they indicated that even when contact had been established with various agencies and statutory financial benefits, or various kinds of other help were technically available, these benefits or help might not be offered at all, or be improperly refused. Social workers are particularly criticized for a considerable variation in enthusiasm for their work with people with the disease, and it is noted that

> The chief factor affecting a patient's receipt of his full entitlement of social-service benefits seemed to be how alert, persistent, and even aggressive the patient and his or her relatives were.
>
> (Elian and Dean 1983: 1,093)

Thus there may be a considerable onus on the person with multiple sclerosis, and/or their family, to undertake their own assessment of their situation and pursue their entitlements, even against the advice of the representatives of the professional agencies whose aims are ostensibly to aid and support them. In this respect the multiplicity of agencies, their relatively parochial areas of concern, and the poor communication between them is likely to produce major difficulties for individuals. This may well be compounded by the progressive and unpredictable nature of the disease in which the speed of provision of financial entitlements, equipment, or services is vital, in order to minimize the risk of that provision being inappropriate to a newly changed condition. As Kerrie says:

> Wishing to be as independent as possible I'm sure that I get aids some months after they would be of positive value. The progressive nature of the condition means that you are never sure how you might be in six months time.

The solution to this kind of problem, as in other areas of life for the person with the disease, is to engage actively in research and experimentation to find the most appropriate pathways through the maze of agencies and associated legislation. However, this also requires energy and commitment – which may be at a premium – as well as a high level of skill and experience, and often other resources, both financial and practical.

In general many of the services available to people with multiple sclerosis, as for people with other disabilities, are 'crisis led', or at the very least individually initiated, rather than systematically or automatically given. As Elian and Dean imply, in these circumstances knowledge, persistence, and aggression are likely to be the most effective lubricants of the system of provision. Patrick indicates some of the problems:

> The greatest help [for the person with multiple sclerosis] is people, but we have to find it out the hard way how to get the most from them. My doctor assumed I knew how to get a walking stick and later a chair but I didn't. He had to make the contacts with the authorities for me. I found a bladder aid once I got the GP to refer me to the 'Appliance Clinic' but would have known nothing about it until told by a friend – education is so vital to folk who cannot put the effort into searching out solutions.

Even when services are supplied after this kind of initiative, it is a personal struggle to hold on to them:

> I began to find out what other help was available to me and

since April 1983 I have had a local authority home-help for three hours a week to do the housework. This is a great boon because she knocks the house into shape and I can ignore the housework. However, I have always felt guilty about accepting this help, not least because of her attitude – she continually tells me about the poor old folk she goes to and they only get one hour a week! If it wasn't for my GP and health visitor insisting that I continue with this help, and my husband insisting that without it the work would not get done, I would give it up, particularly because I feel so fit now. When I was first diagnosed, housework sapped my strength and energy enormously and left nothing for caring for the children, who were and are my top priority. Having a home-help and a child-minder meant that I could survive through till the children's bed-time and might even have some energy left over for my husband – though usually not a lot.

Concern about the potential difficulties of receiving additional services, perhaps by being seen as too demanding, can inhibit those who are, in a sense, already in the system – to the extent that eligibility may not even be tested:

I cannot remember when in 1979 I contacted the social services or particularly what for. All I know is a person did call and arranged for a physiotherapist to give me certain exercises but as luckily at the time I was very mobile and had a steady home life, there was little else they felt they could do. . . . In due course, I had an extra hand-rail fitted to the stairs, and some handles to help up the outside steps. I also now have a home-help, although due to pressures and cutbacks, she is only able to come two hours once a week. . . . I have discovered that should my condition deteriorate there are further facilities available, i.e. a shower seat, an entry phone, etc., but knowing how stretched the social services are at the moment, I have not even enquired what extra help they could offer.

Such a view of the system of provision leads to a perception that services, financial support, or the provision of equipment are not a matter of rights and entitlement, but a matter of fortunate generosity despite – or perhaps because of – the hurdles which have to be overcome in the process of application:

As to the DHSS, I discovered from another sufferer that I could claim both mobility allowance and married woman's non-contributory pension. Both necessitated much form-filling, confirmation from GP, and examinations from independent doctors but I was again one of the lucky ones and receive both. Our car tax is also paid, so this takes some of the strain off Robin. We use the mobility allowance to buy my car and some of the pension to pay for the home-help.

Thus the indications seem to be that whatever the formal structure of support from the many agencies which, in terms of their objectives, would appear to offer help to people with the disease, it is largely through the efforts of the people themselves that any substantial inroads are likely to be made into their needs for services.

One of the problems of seeking the kind of practical or service support that may make life easier practically, is that at each stage in the progression of the disease the need for such support is a clear personal and social indicator of abilities lost. The difficulties of obtaining equipment that is suitable for any particular individual relate partly to the almost infinite gradation of functional problems that may appear at any one time, as well as the unpredictable and unstable physical trajectory of the disease. Therefore life appears to be a continuing round of modifications, adaptations, and 'making do', in which any one solution may be only temporary. Using particular pieces of equipment is also likely to have a 'domino effect' on other equipment or the environment in which the equipment is used. Thus cars or houses used prior to wheelchair acquisition may now be inappropriate, and themselves require modification or change. Richard notes that he

cannot sit in the NHS wheelchair for long. . . . This has been overcome by buying a larger softer chair with a sloping back, which enables me to sit comfortably for long periods. The only snag is that it is too big to go into the converted minivan which we have and is too big to go through the standard door frame.

There is considerable practical (and lateral) thinking that often needs to be undertaken to fit the solution to the personal problems involved. Thus even (or perhaps especially) when equipment is provided through statutory sources, as in the case of Richard above, personal modifications may seem necessary:

the wide high chair provided by the DHSS which can be used for perching, for me . . . proved virtually useless as, on sitting, it was impossible to push back because of weight and rubber feet (necessary I realize for stability). My husband felt sure he could make the chair suitable for my particular problems so, after seeking permission, he took exactly the right amount off to ensure the very useful handles cleared the top of my low work surface. Four new small plastic feet allowed me to push the chair back (on a vinyl tiled floor) and now I would not be able to manage without it. The OT [occupational therapist] was delighted with the result as she had told me she had not found one person who was happy with the chair in its original design.

The broad financial consequences of multiple sclerosis may be as dramatic as the practical problems that arise and need to be solved. Poverty stemming from, or associated with, physical impairment has been found to be common (Blaxter 1976: 89–132). The financial consequences of multiple sclerosis for individuals and their families are difficult to calculate accurately but on any basis appear to be substantial (O'Brien 1987). Marjorie succinctly indicates the interlocking nature of the disease and its disturbing and unpredicted financial consequences for her:

[Three years after my diagnosis] I had a second attack followed by a fall, and a broken arm . . . then I had to stop work. If only I had realized that I should plan financially for the future instead of pressing on. I have now lost all my material possessions, and am just about to move out of my four-bedroom detached house in X to a two-bedroom council flat. . . . I was given no warning of future effects . . . and it would have been very helpful if I could have been prepared for my financial demise.

Marion feels guilty about the effect that losing her own part-time job has had on her husband and on her family's financial position:

Due to excessive tiredness, I decided to give up my job, even though it was only a matter of hours twice a week. However when bills start accumulating and the children need so much, I watch Walter worrying and feel even more guilty, as I am not able to help any more.

At a time when the future is a cause for considerable concern life assurance becomes another problem, in which desperate personal solutions may not turn out the way that had been hoped:

> Another traumatic episode in that year was Gordon's difficulty in getting life insurance. He needed this to get a loan from the building society. After he was refused by two companies I suggested he should lie about his health. I justified this by thinking that the insurance companies were so ignorant that they thought MS was fatal, so they were wrong in refusing life insurance. On the other hand if he died of MS and they found out they would refuse to pay anyway, but we would have our loan and our conscience would be clear. What I did not realize was that insurance companies have a central blacklist of people who have been refused by other companies. So our ruse was discovered. Gordon was carpeted by the insurance executive and I felt very guilty. We did eventually get insurance at enormous expense and excluding cover for death with MS.

The financial solutions available to people with the disease may be limited, largely because income and employment are strongly associated, and it is loss of full-time or part-time employment that is a common consequence of the disease (see Chapter 4). Even so the take-up of available benefits, limited though they are, is low. In Elian and Dean's study somewhere between 10 per cent and 30 per cent of the people with multiple sclerosis they studied appeared to be eligible for allowances or benefits which they were not receiving – and in most cases had not even applied for (1983: 1,092). Radford and Trew note the particular difficulties involved in applying for such benefits (1987: 79).

In summary it seems that despite the catalogue of services which Blaxter noted – all of which were technically available to people with disabilities, including those with multiple sclerosis – people with the disease and others informally helping or caring for them were frequently, indeed usually, thrown back on their own resources.

The infrastructure of informal support – family and friends

Much recent research has indicated the comprehensive nature and the vital significance of what might be called the informal care and support of those with disabilities (Briggs and Oliver 1985). Everyday care is largely in the hands of family and friends for most people with disabilities. This type of care invariably focuses attention on the interpersonal relationships in which the care and support is situated. Blaxter concluded in her study that although

> practical troubles of money, work, daily living [were the ones] that the patients were, in general, most anxious to talk about first . . . it became clear that in a number of cases the problems were largely social – problems of marital relationships and family roles, or alternatively of isolation and loneliness, problems of boredom and lack of social interaction. These were some of the unhappiest people in the sample.
>
> (Blaxter 1976: 196)

Although there is at present limited published evidence of the balance between formal professional support and informal care in relation to people with multiple sclerosis, Elian and Dean's study of service provision for such people strongly suggests that informal care constitutes by far the greater part of the overall provision (1983). It is likely therefore that the social problems that Blaxter locates, particularly in and around family structures for people with all kinds of disabilities, will be just as great in relation to people with multiple sclerosis (Radford and Trew 1987).

Accounts of the nature of informal support for those with multiple sclerosis, both by people with the disease and those in their immediate family, stress the social context of the practical tasks they undertake. This is epitomized in many respects in the idea of the 'being' rather than the 'doing' part of the support for the person with the condition.

'Being there' is important in two senses. First, in order to maintain the continuity of relationships from the past – before the diagnosis, through the present, and into the future. This continuity ensures that the 'fractured biography' (Bury 1982) produced through the disintegration of health, leaves social relationships as intact as is possible. Second, the 'being there' provides an additional resource of energy, and perhaps even a fundamental motivation, for those who are fighting the disease. In this sense stopping its incursions, and especially attempting to roll back the damage already incurred – a formidable and perhaps forlorn personal task – is aided by the mutual meeting of minds. For Carol it is a hard slog through the deserts of the disease, in which the trek is made possible by both the companionship and the pressure of her husband; failure is not on the agenda:

> [After the diagnosis] I had a feeling of worry as to how my husband would react after being married six months and being told your wife has MS. Would he leave me? Could he cope? But then I knew that I didn't have to worry because we are both strong and that all he would do is to chastise me if I gave in . . . and no way was I going to give in to it . . . my husband says we will tackle each problem as and when it comes.

Sally puts forward a slightly more tentative formulation of the same strategy:

> I was greatly helped by my husband and friends . . . [in helping me to realize] that if I could acknowledge the illness, accept it (to a certain extent) and then fight it off, I would be able to forget about it.

Such a strategy, while binding together the partners in a common struggle and providing mutual comfort, has its drawbacks. Bobby considers that the major support his wife has given him has not only led to her problems, but also rebounded on him:

> Needless to say we have fought the disease everyway and are still fighting. I must emphasize that if it were not for the support and assistance my wife has given me all these years, I could not have coped, mentally or physically. In fact I firmly believe that the strain has been greater on her than me, especially as she is not in the best possible health, having suffered a fractured disc in her spine . . . needless to say the worry and strain of this incident brought on another attack of MS in me.

Bobby's predicament emphasizes both the strength and the weakness of this mutually committed approach, which may be used by the parents of people with the disease, as well as by husbands, wives, and partners. The reciprocal support in this situation can be quickly undermined if the health of one or both of the partners deteriorates, or if any other bastion measuring the success of the fight crumbles in the face of the march of time. None the less the early and powerful allegiance of intimate others, whatever the long-term outcome of the relationship, is a bonus compared to a situation where partners melt away early in the face of the disease.

The role of friends appears to be a more problematic one in relation to the level and nature of their support for the person with multiple sclerosis. The restructuring of friendships attendant on physical incapacity produced through the progression of the disease is noted in Cunningham's study (1977: 75–7). As she indicates, the problems partially relate to the potential for the destruction of current relationships, and the difficulty of their replacement by others. As the disease produces disabilities, these may bite into the physical capacities on which some friendships are founded, a particular problem for the young and previously physically active. The basis of mutual support on which such friendships can be sustained must be changed to ensure their viability. However, when the discrepancy between the physical performance of those with multiple sclerosis and friends amongst their contemporaries is less – as in later middle age when a range of incapacitating health problems become more common for all – friendships appear to be more readily kept (M. Z. Davis 1973; Cunningham 1977: 77).

Alternative sources of support? – charitable concerns

The perceived inadequacies of existing services, with the pressure on personal and family resources, and the potential for making common cause amongst people with multiple sclerosis, indicate that organizations and groups outside the formal medical structure might offer considerable support to such people. Indeed chronic diseases in particular are associated with charitable organizations and self-help groups. In relation to those conditions, like multiple sclerosis, which focus attention on a potentially bleak future:

> the existence of self-help groups may represent a sort of lifeline – a link, a bridge into companionship, a sense of belonging which the illness or problem has denied them. It offers a new reference group, a reorientation from gazing on the blank wall of solitude to sharing in a society of likeminded people.
> (McEwen, Martini, and Wilkins 1983: 107)

Such groups have been found by Robinson and Henry to originate – according to the accounts of their members – from three major concerns. First, the failure of existing services, second, the recognition of the value of mutual help, and third, the role of the media in publicizing their case (D. Robinson and Henry 1977: 12). In this discussion evidence of the first two concerns has been clearly documented, and the third is evident in the behaviour of those groups active in relation to multiple sclerosis.

In Chapters 2 and 5, and earlier in this chapter, the perceived failure of the existing services – medical or non-medical – to provide good, satisfactory, or even adequate support for many people with multiple sclerosis in relation to a variety of their needs or wishes has been considered. As McEwen, Martini, and Wilkins indicate, this may be as much because of inability as the unwillingness on the part of the professional individuals or agencies concerned (1983: 109). People with the disease may have certain aims and objectives which differ from those of such individuals or agencies which make it unlikely that all those aims could be professionally met. None the less the gap between expectation and provision is such as to lead to a belief that other ways of organizing existing services should be espoused, or the services should be complemented, or circumvented by a different and more effective mode of provision.

The value of mutual help may be discovered in a number of socially and personally supportive strategies for individuals considered in this analysis. At a more formally organized level such mutual help may be employed to disseminate knowledge about multiple sclerosis, and engage with personal and emotional difficulties attendant on the disease. In addition the mutual help may be employed in distributing information on the disease and giving support for the day-to-day managerial and practical problems which arise. Further and at a more general level, the mutual help may be used to create a broad base of people with the disease to generate funds for activities ranging from the management of personal and practical problems, to developing new research strategies, and seeking appropriate changes of local or national policy and practice.

In making known the perceived inadequacies of existing services, developing remedies to those inadequacies, or establishing alternative or additional services the role of the media is important. They may be used to establish knowledge about the disease in the public mind; to alert others with the disease to the existence of the group; to publicize the group's role and services; to create a sense of solidarity or unity amongst those with the disease; to identify weaknesses in current service provision; to raise funds; and to endeavour to create pressure for change favourable to the group's members and interests.

The broad sets of strategies which could be employed are not mutually exclusive – indeed all three are likely to be linked together. However, the precise strategy followed by such a group, and indeed its basic structure, may depend, as Katz has argued, on other factors. In particular it may depend on the nature and intensity of the group's beliefs and values; on its attitudes towards professional groups and agencies; on the degree to which it supports or rejects the values of the society in which it operates; and on the kind of organizational framework it has (Katz 1979: 491–4).

Not surprisingly given the problematic and – at least for the foreseeable future – intractable condition of multiple sclerosis, there is a diversity of approaches amongst societies associated with the disease. This in turn reflects the diversity of approaches, goals, and interests of people with multiple sclerosis. For some people joining a society is an appropriate indeed natural thing to do following their diagnosis, for mutual support and information, and to help through their own efforts the subjugation of the disease from whose demise they would greatly benefit.

For others the question of whether to join a society at all may be a major decision. In Miles's discussion of the issue (1979) she suggests that becoming a member of a society associated with the disease is in itself limited with the strategy of withdrawal from interaction with the non-multiple-sclerosis community. She argues from her study that this decision indicates a change of self-identity from the community of the 'healthy' to that of the community of the 'ill'. It becomes a decision which as Miles indicates her respondents did not take lightly, and may be reached only after a great deal of thought. For example Jane explains:

Although I knew about the MS branch it was in fact years before I contacted them and began to get involved. Just recently I came to the conclusion that I prefer 'to do' than 'to be done to', and I hope my condition enables me 'to do' for a long time.

Some people with multiple sclerosis may delay joining a voluntary organization associated with the disease – or maintain a very low profile in their contacts – because of their perception that their social and personal identity will be prematurely transformed. They may also feel – at least when their functional problems are slight – that this contact exposes them to others whose more severe disabilities are an unwelcome reminder of the progression of the disease.

The precise reasons why people do or do not join voluntary organizations associated with the disease are still a matter of debate, but are likely to be complex. Which society people join, as well as whether they join any society at all, depends on their own beliefs, the information they seek, and the objectives they are pursuing. It also may depend on the advice they are given, and the resource as well as personal costs and benefits of any action they take.

The diversity of interests amongst people with multiple sclerosis has led to a pattern of societies in Britain with rather different sets of objectives and approaches to meeting the challenge posed by multiple sclerosis. In some respects the key variable is the societies' attitude towards and contact with professional groups and interests – particularly with the medical profession.

One view of the role of the medical profession in relation to multiple sclerosis is that it, and associated medical and other scientists, hold the only key to the future conquest of the disease. In this view the special scientific expertise of clinicians and medical scientists not only gives them privileged access to the techniques needed for research and therapy, but – just as important – also places them in a uniquely informed position to decide priorities. For their realization, these medical priorities need the support and funding by people with multiple sclerosis, their families, and other interested parties who, in the process, can gain from such support, as well as the mutual aid offered by participating in this way. The Multiple Sclerosis Society, the largest society associated with the disease in the United Kingdom, might be considered to be linked with this approach, as well as other multiple sclerosis societies in many other countries throughout the world, linked together through the International Federation of Multiple Sclerosis Societies.

The organization of these societies, although different in detail, follows the general model adopted by the British Multiple Sclerosis Society, and that in the USA. Although each of these two societies has a governing body containing elected lay representatives which formally decides the policy of the society, in many respects the most important advice comes from the relevant medical committee, in Britain the Medical Research Advisory Committee. This committee

> composed of research scientists and specialists in neurology [recommends] which lines of research are worth pursuing and advise[s] the Society on media reports of 'breakthroughs', and on the many claims of treatments and cures in MS. This committee makes sure that the MS Society spends its money wisely and that it is kept up to date on all aspects of MS.
>
> (Burnfield 1985: 177)

In relation to medical matters it is anticipated that those with the disease in the society would offer support and resources to the work of this committee, and follows its authoritative advice on the status of putative therapies and other related matters. Other aspects of the society's work, including fund-raising and what might be generally termed welfare activities, are co-ordinated by other staff and lay members of the society in a voluntary capacity with relevant professional advice.

As with medical matters, the policy of the society in welfare and other issues of concern is established by the governing body and implemented through the network of branches. However, within this policy, branches almost entirely managed and run by volunteers may engage in a variable mixture of fund-raising, social meetings, practical help and advice, personal support, and consultation with other organizations and agencies. One such branch

> meets regularly each month in a friendly local pub and the members enjoy a drink together, play games, and occasionally have talks and discussions with subjects which may or may not be related to MS. As well as this the branch publicizes itself in the local press, collects money on flag days, and goes in for a variety of fund-raising activities. There is also an MS CRACK group for the younger members who may wish to talk together, to share their problems, and find solutions.
>
> (Burnfield 1985: 178)

Burnfield goes on to indicate that other branches may spend less of their time in social meetings and more in fund-raising and practical support through, for example, day centres and some financial assistance for their members, or help for holiday breaks.

Primarily therefore at branch level the Multiple Sclerosis Society in the United Kingdom is engaged in personal, social, and practical assistance for those with the disease, together with fundraising for the society's research and other activities. Many people with multiple sclerosis, and their families, find this pattern both very helpful and personally supportive, and soon become actively involved, as Joy indicates:

A few months after my suspicions of my MS had been confirmed it became apparent that unlike Karen [a girl she had seen come in hospital unable to walk, and then walk out again] I was not going to walk again. It was then the depression set in. I telephoned Karen and told her how I felt, and how utterly devastated my husband was. I was encouraged by her to join the local branch of the MS society, and despite reservations and advice against this move, I felt they had to do something, and talk to someone who understood. Joining the local branch of the MS Society proved to be the best move I had made for years. I made many new friends and renewed my friendship with Karen. I became an active member and served on the committee for some years, only relinquishing this when manoeuvring myself in and out of the car became more difficult.

Others also find the concern of others through the medium of the society both a surprise and a support, as Barbara comments, when after a relapse she

was amazed at the flowers, cards, and visits I had from friends in the [MS] Society. The main thing about our society is the way that everyone feels for each other. If one member is ill, everyone is anxious.

However, for some people with multiple sclerosis, the kind of support represented in the philosophy and activities of the society is considered personally inappropriate. They feel they want more active involvement in the management of their disease through direct control of the direction and implementation of medical policy and practice. This leads to a second view of the relationship between people with multiple sclerosis and those professions medically associated with its management. This approach suggests that, although the key to the conquest of the disease lies with the medical profession and medical scientists, their priorities and objectives need supplementing and guiding (perhaps even directing) by those with the disease whose priorities and ideas may be based on different perspectives. In this case the support and funding is of a kind where priorities may be decided in effect by those outside the medical profession – albeit after consultation with clinicians and medical scientists – although subsequent research and practice may take place within that medical domain. ARMS (Action for Research into Multiple Sclerosis) might be considered to be associated with this approach.

The personal philosophy which might be linked with this view is expressed with some vigour by Barry:

> Disabled people can too easily be made to feel useless. The development of their personal creativity could play an important part in overcoming this. Here, I must say, some organizations can be positively harmful in that they rob the disabled person of much of the control of his or her own life. This is where the 'self-help' approach is so vitally important. I now understand how 'do-gooding' can be a real disservice to those trying to retain their pride, independence, and individuality. Yes, we all need help, but encouraging, strengthening help, not the kind that robs us of dignity. One local branch of a well-known society offered to entertain me with magicians and trips to the zoo – this whilst I was still teaching! I soon realized that some of those involved with this branch wanted me to be a totally passive recipient of their good works and charity. No thank you! It still infuriates me that this same society branch sends me a £5 gift voucher each Christmas, money that could be channelled to individual sufferers in real need, or for valuable research. Having MS shouldn't entitle me to such handouts if I do not really need them. People give generously to these societies. The money should be spent wisely. This is why, until recently, I had been so pleased with ARMS, though our own local branch has suffered from the 'do-gooding' syndrome with a few non-sufferers taking over the group without any real commitment. It was obvious that they wanted those with the disease to sit back and be good, quiet children. It is such a difficult problem, as one doesn't want to hurt people, but if only they realized the harm that they do. There are, thank goodness, marvellous, unselfish, genuine helpers, working very hard with

the disabled. Infuriatingly though, there are many others who feel the disabled should stay silent and accept every half-hearted, gratitude-seeking and deadening attempt to 'help'.

Barry's account fuses a number of themes common to those who press for a more independent and active role in relation to their multiple sclerosis. They believe that they are the best judge of their interests, medical as well as personal or social, and reject what they deem to be the misguided approach of others, whether they be professionals or, in Barry's case, 'non-sufferers'.

ARMS, despite Barry's caveat about a particular branch, seems broadly to embody his beliefs about how those with multiple sclerosis should be treated. ARMS was founded in 1974 – nearly twenty-five years after the Multiple Sclerosis Society – by a small group of people with the disease and their relatives specifically to generate a new momentum for research into multiple sclerosis from outside the established medical approach. Membership was restricted to people with the disease or those immediately caring for them. Unlike the Multiple Sclerosis Society, which differentiated between those areas subject to proper and authoritative medical advice, and other areas more amenable to lay judgement, ARMS in effect fused these two areas through emphasizing the key policy-making role of people with multiple sclerosis and their families in establishing priorities in all matters relating to the disease.

As might be expected, given the special weight attached to the role of people with the disease and their families at all levels of decision-making, there has until recently been less centralized organization of the branches in ARMS than in the Multiple Sclerosis Society. The activities of the branches have been diverse but based on a very different approach from that of the Society. They have generally not been established specifically for social or fund-raising objectives, or for practical support for people's everyday lives – although all three activities may be found. Almost all of the branches have been established for the explicit purpose of managing multiple sclerosis through the use of various therapies, re-emphasizing the self-help component of ARMS outside the domain and site of conventional medical practice. Currently the majority of the branches have facilities for hyperbaric oxygen, and many offer physiotherapy, nutrition, or counselling advice.

Although some branches of ARMS were formed early in the

life of the organization, many more branches have been formed in the last four years on a wave of enthusiasm by people with the disease for hyperbaric oxygen therapy. This therapy, which involves the use of pressurized chambers in which oxygen is piped through masks to those in the chamber, gained great support amongst people with multiple sclerosis following early promising research results, and following people's own experience with the therapy. After further clinical trials conventional medical opinion is now that hyperbaric oxygen has little or no place in the management of the disease. None the less it is still an important focus of the activities of many ARMS branches, with the use of the therapy supported by other doctors and medical scientists who believe that standard clinical trials have not tested and cannot fully test the efficacy of hyperbaric oxygen.

The use by ARMS of managerial strategies like diet, dietary supplements, and more recently hyperbaric oxygen therapy, particularly where that use has been at variance with conventional medical opinion, has led to considerable differences of opinion between ARMS and the Multiple Sclerosis Society. This conflict may also have been partly centred on a general concern over members, funds, and influence, as well as on rather different views about the nature, extent, and response to medical authority, which the role of hyperbaric oxygen therapy crystallized. This therapy, despite conventional medical scepticism about its use, and therefore discouragement from the Multiple Sclerosis Society, enticed some people from the society to try it, as demonstrated in Brian's case – moreover with the help of the local MSS branch:

[My first contact with MS Society was after my wife's serious MS attack] . . . I know the name of the chairman of the nearby MS Society and I wrote to him. He was very supportive but I did not get his phone-call in reply to my letter until after Christmas. . . . [then after a lengthy hospital stay for his wife] we scaled down our involvement in local groups and became more and more involved with the MS Society. We set up a local branch and I was the first chairman. . . . [Brian then decided he must have HBO therapy for his wife, and had to buy a chamber because of the distance they had to travel for the therapy] The chamber cost £6,500 . . . the MS Society of which we are both prominent members does not approve of the treatment. Despite this the local branch, which is autonomous moneywise, gave some financial support towards it.

The relationship between these two societies – at an organizational level – has been complex and fragile largely because of different attitudes towards the role of established medical opinion, in addition to other factors.

However, despite the differences in approach between the two organizations, there are complementary aspects to their work. In research the Multiple Sclerosis Society engages in a great deal of basic scientific work, while ARMS with its more limited resources concentrates on techniques and strategies of immediate managerial significance. The two organizations have complementary interests in the social, personal, and employment consequences of the disease, and on the provision of better services to alleviate some of its effects.

For individuals, as Rosemary indicates above, an eclectic approach to the use of the two organizations and their facilities and benefits may often be used. Whatever the state of relations between the two charities, many people belong to both, as Burnfield notes (1985: 182). Others may engage in the kind of experimentation discussed in Chapter 5 to try and find the organization that is right for them, as Norman describes:

From then [when he was diagnosed] I started reading more and writing to both societies. I first joined the MS Society, and although their literature gave hope, their monthly bulletins seemed to be for the truly disabled people; this didn't give me any hope. I found the ARMS format much more geared to my interests. ARMS gave me a lot of help; it gave me a regime to follow.

John on the contrary found the MS Society provided the support that he wanted:

After the diagnosis I felt that I wanted to follow the best medical advice I could, and after reading both what the MS Society and ARMS had to offer, it seemed to me that the main thing I could do was to support the medical researchers through joining and fund-raising for my local MS Society – it is through them a cure will come in the end.

In conclusion, the use of organizations such as the Multiple

Sclerosis Society and ARMS is an important feature of many people's lives. They provide a means of focusing hope, anger, desperation, needs for companionship in a common situation, a wish to help others, a search for practical advice, and many other concerns which cannot easily be met in the intimacy of family life, or in the colder world of professional medicine.

Supporting those with multiple sclerosis and their families

The indications are that there is an enormous catalogue of unmet medical, practical, personal, and social need amongst those with multiple sclerosis and their families. The emphasis of medical services, especially in hospitals, has continued to be on the diagnosis of the condition rather than on the alleviation or management of symptoms, or the rehabilitation of people with the disease. Even in the area of diagnosis where the concentration of much specialist energy is apparent, the experience of patients has not on the whole been positive, or modestly satisfactory. In the community, the diversity of services, their different objectives and procedures and their problematic co-ordination, places the onus on the person with the condition and their family to seek out, find, and use such services and support as they can. The system of formal health care is patently not working, at least for most people with multiple sclerosis, for it requires considerable personal resources of energy in addition to skill and experience in using services which themselves are in short supply. Thus support is centred on the informal environment of the person, occasional interventions from professional help, often the use of organizations associated with the disease, and whatever sources of aid can be mustered from family and friends. In these circumstances practical support and hope must be maintained in a variety of ways to retain a viable and rewarding life.

Chapter seven

Making sense of the future: maintaining faith and hope

Multiple sclerosis presents a common dilemma for all who come into contact with it. For the person with the disease and their families, as well as clinicians and medical scientists, the puzzle presented by its onset, course, and consequences leads to a diverse array of attempted solutions to that puzzle. Each one of these attempted solutions, whether it is tried scientifically in the laboratory or personally in the home, is experimental in the sense of trying to find some way of understanding and controlling the disease and its effects. All of those involved in this search have their own particular sets of objectives about what they would like to achieve, which sometimes coincide and sometimes conflict, as the disease affects so many aspects of the lives of those bound up professionally and personally with it.

However, underlying much of the experience of multiple sclerosis is a concern for the future, and the need to maintain a realistic sense of hope. For the individual the problem is to try not only to avoid the further bodily ravages of what is, after all, medically recognized as a progressive condition, but also even more importantly to avoid damage to the integrity of the self. In the same way, for families and friends it is a question of trying to maintain the integrity of relationships in the light of intrusion of the disease. For clinicians it is a question of maintaining positive relationships with their patients when their resources, both personal and medical, are severely stretched. For medical scientists it is a question of maintaining a scientific approach to the disease in the light of the special problems posed by research into multiple sclerosis and in the knowledge of the hopes and expectations of others.

Medicine and medical research as a source of hope

The role of medicine and medical research is particularly important as a source of hope and promise for the future both for those with the disease and doctors and medical scientists themselves. Thus whatever the current problems which may be experienced between people with multiple sclerosis and their doctors, and whatever disappointments may arise in the scientific search for control of the disease, the power and promise of medicine is such that hope in the future of medical success may be sustained.

Given the multiplicity of theories about the possible causes of multiple sclerosis the search for a means of scientifically containing the disease proceeds on a very broad front. Indeed this wide-ranging and often fiercely competitive effort is both a spur to the medical scientists involved, and a considerable consolation to those with multiple sclerosis. One of the main ways that hope can be sustained in medical science is by a belief in the global scale of the research effort, and the great variety of therapies and techniques which might be being clinically tested – all, or some of which, could work. Even if one apparently promising therapy falls by the wayside, another could be resurrected in its place. There is always the perceived possibility of something 'about to happen', in relation to which Abby hopes she could 'sort the wheat from the chaff', as she puts it:

> I have recently taken a keen interest in research into MS and any new developments in diagnosis and treatment. I am sceptical about the benefits of HBO but am hopeful that the new magnetic resonance imaging scanners being used will enable the effects of therapy of any sort to be evaluated scientifically. I belong both to ARMS and the MS Society and do a small amount of fund-raising for both. I read everything I can lay my hands on which may have a bearing on the subject, and I hope my scientific and medical training enables me to sort the wheat from the chaff.

Such an approach as that which Abby adopts can lift people's vision from the problematic and practical plane of their present troubles to the more promising plane of future medical success, and thereby generates hope. Moreover because 'the future' is such an indeterminate concept which can be compressed to be very near the present and yet expanded to be very far away, all –

whether people with the disease or medical scientists – can use this pliability to keep their beliefs and hopes intact. It seems likely that the concept of 'the future' in relation to the promise of medicine is further away for doctors and medical scientists, than it is for people with the disease – although it may not be helpful for either party to acknowledge that this is in fact the case. Wilfred emphasizes the instant hopes of many people with multiple sclerosis:

> I never give up hope that some dramatic breakthrough will be made in the treatment of diseases of the nervous system, as there has been in other complaints considered incurable, that respond to modern drugs or techniques and give hope to young victims that they will not be confined to a wheelchair and have to rely on help for many of the 'things' that we are only too pleased when a baby grows [up that it does] for itself.

As one of those 'young victims' Andrea expresses a similar view:

> I look forward with hope that a cure may be found and am thankful that I don't seem to have deteriorated since diagnosis. I hope I will go along the same for years or until the cure is found. In the mean time I will continue with my yoga and diet and keep myself as busy and interested in life as possible.

Participation in the enterprise of medical research itself may be a way of sustaining these hopes in a more active way. With the large number of clinical trials, and medical research being undertaken on various potential therapies (see Robinson 1987b) it is a distinct possibility that people, particularly in the earlier stages of the disease, may have the opportunity of being part of the medical research process. Such participation may bring hopes of the possibility of personal benefit, the provision of special medical care, the possibility of helping others indirectly, and more broadly the opportunity to feel part of a team engaged in medical research. Kerry's account provides a flavour of the hopes that such participation can provide:

> I went to see the doctor at the hospital and he offered me a place in a trial paid for by the MRC [Medical Research Council]. . . . It wasn't going to do me any harm and it might do me some good. . . . I jumped at the idea. . . . I was called

to the hospital . . . during the first three days we met the team
. . . the same doctor would set up the drips each morning and
because I had small deep veins he developed a real hang-up
about mine. I used to make him sit on my bed and relax
completely before attempting to get the needle in! We all got
to know each other very well. . . . I still continued to improve
whilst I was in there and came home only with a walking stick,
fully convinced that the treatment had worked.

Ultimately Kerry's hopes ended in disappointment from this
experience, for she got worse again, but none the less she still
expressed the wish to participate in other research. For her, hopes
raised about the promise of future research which might still lead
to personal and dramatic improvements overrode the failure of
her expectations on this occasion. However, others, after a series
of perceived disappointments after being let down by the demise
of 'dramatic breakthroughs', can take a much more circumspect
view and espouse the virtues of careful, steady, and long-term
research, as well as the virtues of what Geoff calls a more holistic
approach:

> The last two years have found me increasingly concerned at
> the time and money that ARMS is giving to the HBO
> treatment centres, as I am not convinced of their long-term
> use. Of course this treatment must be carefully examined
> and nurtured, but it seems to have taken so much of ARMS
> commitment. I believe that any long-lasting control and
> improvement of the disease needs patient, time-consuming
> hard work, not instant panaceas. This is why I am so much
> in favour of the holistic 'diet and exercise' approach. It seems
> an eminently sensible way to real progress and I hope ARMS
> will not lose sight of this. Also there are many promising
> avenues of research into the cause, nature, and prevention
> of the disease. These need constant and adequate funding.
> ARMS must be very sure that the HBO chambers are not
> wheel-less 'band-wagons' racing down disappointing,
> expensive culs-de-sac.

Of course in the search for a cure – or a means of effective
management – for multiple sclerosis there have been many possibilities which have been explored. Some of these possibilities have
had very serious side-effects, as well as proving even more costly

than HBO. In the process of the personal assessment of different kinds of therapies no doubt many with multiple sclerosis would say that culs-de-sac for some are open roads for others. This is largely because the practice of medical science in relation to multiple sclerosis is not always uniform and agreed. Given the range of possible causes (and hence therapies) for the disease there are always likely to be disagreements amongst medical scientists in different sub-specialities about the nature and effectiveness of research into and the management of multiple sclerosis. These disagreements generate hope, as well as frustration, because they produce the possibility of new, exciting, and lateral approaches to the problem of the disease.

Hope in medical science is maintained for many people because the possible future production of a cure – remote though it might technically be – is set against what appears to be almost certain bodily decline. In this equation it may appear to people with the disease that they have little or nothing to lose from such faith in medical science, for even if the hoped-for cure is not produced, the faith itself may be an important element in sustaining their daily life. In any case being a party, even a junior and distant one, to the international medical effort to conquer the disease, provides an avenue through which that effort and its successes and failures can, in a sense, be shared by everyone.

Knowledge as the basis of hope

The possible congruence of hopes, expectations, and interests between the person with multiple sclerosis and the medical scientist explored in the discussion above – primarily through the support of the work of medical scientists – is only one of a number of ways in which people with disease manage their futures. For some in the quest for control of their multiple sclerosis, knowledge about the disease provides the personal power they feel can change their lives. This quest is based on acquiring and personally using information from doctors, medical scientists, and others, rather than directly contributing, through research involvement or fund-raising, to it. As Emma puts it:

> I decided to find out as much about MS as a layman could understand. I needed to find out what it was all about – either it took over me, or I fought it.

Or as Nathan notes:

> I must say that I had to find out all the information for myself but having done so I found this has made me feel much more confident and secure for the future than in the first days after the diagnosis when I found that I had a disease I hadn't even heard of.

An avaricious search for information appears to be a frequent reaction to the presence of multiple sclerosis for many throughout life with the disease. 'Information' is seen as a pathway – perhaps an expressway – to individual understanding and control of the disease. The disease to which the information relates is not the disease in general, it is *their* disease. This approach is different from, although it may be complementary to, faith in the role of medicine and medical science.

Although it may be the case that people with the disease and their families seek some broad knowledge about the condition, it often appears that the information is required to answer specific and very pressing questions, as in Jill's case:

> I calmed down [after being told the diagnosis], then went to the library to try and find out all I could about MS. I found out that having MS does not mean dying within a few months and I was very relieved when I had done a lot of reading about it. I felt that I could cope with the disease, a sense of acceptance and a desire to carry on as long as possible.

Or for Julie:

> It was only through my own reading and research that I gradually found out that it was quite possible that I wasn't going to end up in a wheelchair. Hope is vital, even if misplaced.

Such needs for specific information to dispel fears, and to enable the evaluation of how best to manage personal futures, is likely to occur throughout life with the disease. In this relation to these needs two of the major concerns about information provided by doctors have been first that it may be imprecise and general (Tuckett *et al.* 1985: 36–7), and second that it may be unrelated to patients' objectives.

It is likely therefore that the use and transformation of medically sponsored information into personally meaningful knowledge will take place outside a formal medical context; perhaps even outside the public domain altogether, as Cornwell (1985) puts it. In this case making sense of and creating hope out of information given in that medical context becomes a personal affair.

None the less there may be other allies, even if individual doctors may not be able to (or capable of) dealing with the agendas of people with multiple sclerosis themselves. The organizations concerned with the disease may act as important mediators in the process of turning medical information into personally digestible and relevant knowledge. Gavin sees this as one amongst a number of possibilities:

> a doctor should also be able to give details of all that is available to help, i.e. the address of societies, the titles of books and literature, and where to find it. [Also] where to find out about diets that might help, because I found that after being told I had MS I was left to my own devices and the doctors had no more interest in me.

In this context the interpretation of and support for the very diverse range of strategies, that people may wish to pursue in and through the knowledge they gain, is likely to be easier for those organizations which can take clear account of the personal aims and objectives of people with the disease, as much as those of the medical profession. For above all the use of information by people with the disease is set in the framework of personal rather than medical control, and set in personally rescuing the self from the loss of identity indicated by Charmaz (1983). It is also set in the framework of faith and hope, concepts not easy for doctors to articulate in general, and particularly not easy to articulate in relation to this disease.

Finding hope in the supernatural

Faith in the supernatural ordering of events and circumstances, particularly in the understanding of the meaning of multiple sclerosis and the problems it brings in its train, is a not unexpected consequence for some in the absence of other commonly accepted and viable explanations of the disease, and in the absence of a medically endorsed cure.

Even amongst those whose medical knowledge may give them privileged access to a range of scientific information about the disease there may be an attempt to explain and come to terms with their situation through considering the role of supernatural events. Burnfield discusses the way that he has sought to understand his situation as a doctor with multiple sclerosis using supernatural terminology:

> there is a more positive aspect to the sick doctor: a healer who has personally experienced the grip of the gods and the unfairness of fate can be a healer with increased powers. Contact with the gods, however painful, may offer us an experience that profoundly alters the way we see things and the way we live our lives.

and later

> I have become very familiar with many of the devils that inhabit my particular hell.
> Meeting the devils and finding a path through the forest of life is a universal experience, for this is a journey that we all make. For me, MS has been a major devil.
>
> (Burnfield 1985: 169)

It is important to separate the idea of a divine or supernatural *cause* for the disease, from the idea of a divine or supernatural *purpose* for the person with the disease after onset. These two features can in their turn be separated from the support sought supernaturally to forbear the trials which multiple sclerosis brings with it. There is little evidence that people with multiple sclerosis attribute the cause of their disease directly to divine intervention. However, finding a divine purpose in the nature and consequences of the disease is a way of making sense of the events that have happened. For Freda it is a belief that is beyond her understanding but none the less profoundly important to her:

> I feel very strongly that we go through problems and suffering and that 'God', Buddha, Muhammad – the Creator – has his reasons. We suffer for a purpose – we cannot always see why – many who are paralysed will say 'That's OK for her' and I see their point. I do not know why I have this faith with no name, this belief. Why do babies die? Why do people go on living when they want to die? There is a reason beyond our reasoning.

Karen links her belief about the divine purpose for her suffering with requests for support, and a simultaneous hope that medical science and faith working together will produce an answer:

> There are plenty of people worse than me and I pray for them. I have great faith in God and believe there is a reason for my suffering. I will probably never know what that reason is, but I pray hard for others like me, our carers, family, and friends. I pray the researchers will soon find a cure for multiple sclerosis.

Some people undergo a complete transformation in their lives through a conversion experience in which their multiple sclerosis appears to be considered an advantage to their lives rather than a problem. However it seems that in John's case he is having difficulty carrying his wife with him on his religious journey:

> In many ways I am glad to have weak legs because it makes me rely on God and his strength. I feel that, as St Paul said, 'When I am weak I am strong'. I have had some wonderful and miraculous answers to prayer. God certainly moves in mysterious ways and it is a constant joy to me the way he controls and organizes things for me, often in surprising ways. When I look back I can see how he has helped and guided me. . . .
>
> Yes, I accept that I have MS, but I have given control of it to God and I believe he can completely heal me. I have been greatly encouraged to hear of cases of MS which have been completely healed in the last year or two – people in wheelchairs who are now completely fit and with no trace of MS. . . .
>
> My wife, who is a church organist, is not yet a Christian, and suffers I think from fear of this disease, although she doesn't like to talk about it. She takes the attitude, 'Think positive. Ignore it and it might go away'. This is contradictory to the Christian view and I accept the disease and am happy to fight it head on in the strength of Christ. It is a spiritual battle for me but many symptoms have disappeared through prayer. One day my wife will feel as I do and we will be able to deal with this together.

As if in response to John's committed view, Harold introduces a note of profound scepticism about his kind of approach, while at the same time finding an earthly purpose of his own:

I [have] decided to thump anyone who tries to tell me that there is some 'divine' purpose in my being struck down – that I was not one of God's chosen few who were making the supreme sacrifice, but I did feel that there was some other purpose, at that time I didn't know what it was – It wasn't until I obtained by BA [university degree] that I discovered that I was uniquely qualified to try and help other disabled people and not just those with MS.

Overall it seems likely that the most common approach to the use of religious faith lies in seeking support through the perceived personal benefits of prayer on the one hand, and social participation in the community of people created in and through church life. Others may however feel that supernatural ideas, and ways of understanding their situation, do not require the acknowledgement of a particular personal religious faith, while those like Harold translate the perceived meaning and purpose of their disease into more earthly channels.

Facing the future through social relationships

A major theme of this discussion has been the interlocking nature of the worlds of those individuals with the disease and those who are members of their family and friends. Faith in the friendship and support of others is an important component of the decreasing physical performance often consequent on the progress of the disease. One response to the disease is to re-evaluate what is seen as the core of social and family relationships to reveal their essence, which may be 'what life is all about', as in Jan's case who wanted to

spend as much time with the children as I could so they could have as near normal a life as possible. It also made me stop and think what life is all about. I appreciated just sitting and watching the children play.

For others the camera of the disease photographs their relationships in an almost unbearably sharp focus. Their faith and trust in, as well as their dependence on, their partners have become critical to their lives, although they may wish additional things as well:

I'd hope to be the one to 'go' first; I couldn't bear life without my husband, his support, understanding, encouragement, and praise of the things that I do. I'd hate my eyesight to fail, seeing my granddaughter grow up, flowers, birds coming for the bread I put out, and TV of course, etc., that I can still make use of my arms and that I won't be a burden to anyone or in a 'home'. I'd like to see a cure for MS, or to be told what causes the illness. To be able to do all I can now, even if it's slower than my 'normal' speed.

The support of such relationships where there is a partner with multiple sclerosis has become a major issue to those concerned with the provision of community services in recent years, not least to try and ensure that the pressures on these relationships do not undermine the faith their members place in them. Although that concern has not been effectively operationalized into a network of professional emotional support, there are the beginnings of such a system in some areas in the USA (Marsh, Ellison, and Strite 1983), and ARMS (Action for Research into Multiple Sclerosis) in Britain has begun to establish counselling services for families as well as people with the disease.

As was extensively discussed in Chapter 4 social relationships in general, and family relationships in particular, are a vital part of the terrain over which the battle with the disease is fought. Faith and trust in those relationships for physical, personal, and social reasons are important components in maintaining a sense of hope for the future with multiple sclerosis at its centre.

Making personal sense of the future

In relation to the disease faith in oneself may be the key, in the last analysis, to keeping an intact identity. This faith may well be associated with the degree to which individuals feel themselves drowned by their disabilities, or have the capacity to rise above them, and feel able in some sense to control their effects on the personally important aspects of life.

In Wright's conceptualization coping and succumbing represent polarized ways of personally dealing with disabilities. Those who *cope* have an active view of their role; they conceive of areas of life in which they can participate as worthwhile; they emphasize what they can do; negative aspects of the disability are deemed to be containable; they seek to adapt their environment, both social and physical, to make it more supportive; and they make value changes to be able to live with their limitations. Those who *succumb* emphasize what they cannot do; they see themselves as passive; as having few areas of life in which they can feel they can participate valuably; the negative aspects of the disability are emphasized and seen as particularly damaging; the only solutions to their problems are seen as prevention and cure; and they either resign themselves to their disability or act as if it does not exist (Wright 1983: 195).

The dichotomy of coping and succumbing – or fighting and accepting as it might be described by people with the disease – is one which is a familiar characterization of behaviour in relation to illness or disability. Succumbing might be seen by many with multiple sclerosis as losing out to the disease, indeed as resulting in the loss of self-identity as discussed by Charmaz (1983). Thus coping tends to be by far the most highly valued strategy. It is an active, vigorous, and enabling idea. This combination is illustrated in what Roger says:

> OK you have got MS – it won't go away so get on with your life. . . . I never hid from anyone what I had and my attitude was – if they know they won't keep saying to me, 'What's the matter with your leg?' I don't want sympathy from anyone, or anyone to feel sorry for me. I have a positive attitude – can and I will. . . . Lots of things I can do. . . . I suppose I have got on top of it because friends say 'You are always cheerful'.

Fighting the disease can be both full of hope – generating some faith in personal futures – and yet be realistic and grounded in the struggles of the present. That is it allows the accomplishment of the necessary arduous and practical tasks of daily living, while preserving the possibility of positive redress to the present disabled state. It may also be a particularly apposite strategy in a situation where further physical degeneration is probable but unpredictable. If no one knows the factors which lead to or inhibit this uncertain progression, who is to say whether 'fighting the disease' might not be one of the marginal factors inhibiting future physical deterioration? In any case even if this hoped-for result does not materialize, the psychological and social bonus of perceived control over other life events may be such as to allow the strategy to be continued. In this setting faith and hope may continue to triumph over the experience of the harsh personal world with multiple sclerosis embodied in it.

References

Acheson, E. D. (1985) 'The epidemiology of multiple sclerosis', in
W. B. Matthews, E. D. Acheson, J. R. Batchelor, and R. O.
Weller, *McAlpine's Multiple Sclerosis*, Edinburgh: Churchill
Livingstone.

Alaszewski, A. (1979) 'Rehabilitation, the remedial therapy professions
and social policy', *Social Science and Medicine*, 431–43.

Alter, M. (1972) 'The distribution of multiple sclerosis and
environmental sanitation', in U. Leibowitz (ed.) *Progress in Multiple
Sclerosis Research and Treatment*, New York: Academic Press.

Alter, M. (1983) 'Current medical treatment of multiple sclerosis',
Clinical Therapeutics 5: 455–60.

Alter, M., Leibowitz, U., and Speer, J. (1966) 'Risk of multiple sclerosis
related at age of immigration to Israel', *Archives of Neurology* 15:
234–7.

Alter, M., Yamoor, M., and Harshe, M. (1974) 'Multiple sclerosis and
nutrition', *Archives of Neurology* 31: 267–72.

Anderson, J. A. D., Buck, C., Danaher, K., and Fry, J. (1977) 'Users
and non-users of doctors – implications for self-care', *Journal of
Royal College of General Practitioners* 155–9.

Baretz, R. M. and Stephenson, G. R. (1981) 'Emotional responses to
multiple sclerosis', *Psychosomatics* 22: 117–27.

Batchelor, J. R. (1985) 'Immunological and genetic aspects of multiple
sclerosis', in W. B. Matthews, E. D. Acheson, J. R. Batchelor, and
R. O. Weller, *McAlpine's Multiple Sclerosis*, Edinburgh: Churchill
Livingstone.

Bates, D. (1987) 'Dietary supplementation in multiple sclerosis', in
F. C. Rose, and R. Jones (eds) *Multiple Sclerosis*, London: J.
Libbey.

Baum, H. M. and Rothschild, B. B. (1981) 'The incidence and
prevalence of reported multiple sclerosis', *Annals of Neurology* 10:
420–8.

Beck, R. P., Warren, E. G., and Whitman, P. (1981) 'Urodynamic
studies in female patients with MS', *American Journal of Obstetrics
and Gynecology* 139(3): 273–6.

Beukelman, D. R., Kraft, G. H., and Freal, J. (1985) 'Expressive communication disorders in persons with multiple sclerosis: a survey', *Archives of Physical Medicine and Rehabilitation* 66: 675–6.

Birrer, C. (1979) *Multiple Sclerosis: A Personal View*, Springfield, Ill: Charles C. Thomas.

Blaxter, M. (1976) *The Meaning of Disability: A Sociological Study of Impairment*, London: Heinemann.

Bloor, M. and Horobin, G. (1975) 'Conflict and conflict resolution in doctor–patient interactions', in C. Cox and A. Meade (eds) *A Sociology of Medical Practice*, London: Collier-Macmillan.

Briggs, A. and Oliver, J. (1985) *Caring: Experiences of Looking After Disabled Relatives*, London: Routledge & Kegan Paul.

Brown, S. and Davis, T. K. (1922) 'The mental symptoms of multiple sclerosis', *Archives of Neurology and Psychiatry* 7: 629.

Burnfield, A. (1985) *Multiple Sclerosis: A Personal Exploration*, London: Souvenir Press.

Bury, M. (1982) 'Chronic illness as biographical disruption', *Sociology of Health and Illness* 4(2): 167–82.

Campling, J. (1981) *Images of Ourselves: Women with Disabilities Talking*, London: Routledge & Kegan Paul.

Cassell, E. J. (1976) 'Disease as an "It": Concepts of disease revealed by patients' presentation of symptoms', *Social Science and Medicine* 10: 143–6.

Charmaz, K. (1983) 'Loss of self: a fundamental form of suffering in the chronically ill', *Sociology of Health and Illness* 5: 168–95.

Clark, V. A., Detels, R., Visscher, B. R., Valdiviezo, N. L., Malmgren, R. M., and Dudley, J. P. (1982) 'Factors associated with a malignant course of multiple sclerosis', *Journal of the American Medical Association* 20 August: 856–60.

Cleeland, C. S., Matthews, C. G., and Hopper, C. L. (1970) 'MMPI profiles in exacerbation and remission of multiple sclerosis', *Psychological Reports* 27: 273–4.

Clifford, D. B., and Trotter, J. L. (1984) 'Pain in multiple sclerosis', *Archives of Neurology* 41: 1,270–2.

Comaroff, J. (1976) 'Communicating information about non-fatal illness', *Sociological Review* 24: 269–90.

Compston, A. (1987a) 'Selection of patients for trials', *Neuroepidemiology* 6: 34–9.

Compston, A. (1987b) 'Can the course of multiple sclerosis be predicted?', in C. P. Warian and J. S. Garfield (eds) *More Dilemmas in Neurology*, Edinburgh: Churchill Livingstone.

Confavereux, C., Aimard, G., and Devic, M. (1980) 'Course and prognosis of multiple sclerosis assessed by computerized data processing of 349 patients', *Brain* 103: 281–300.

Cornwell, J. (1985) *Hard-earned Lives: Accounts of Health and Illness from East London*, London: Tavistock.

Cottrell, S. S., and Wilson, S. A. (1926) 'The affective symptomatology of multiple sclerosis', *Journal of Neurology and Psychopathology* 7: 1–30.

References

Cunningham, D. J. (1977) *Stigma and Social Isolation: Self-Perceived Problems of a Group of Multiple Sclerosis Sufferers*, report no. 27, Health Services Research Unit, Centre for Research in the Social Sciences, University of Kent, Canterbury.

Davidson, D. L. W. (1987) 'Supplementary hyperbaric oxygen therapy for multiple sclerosis', in F. C. Rose and R. Jones (eds) *Multiple Sclerosis*, London: J. Libbey.

Davis, F. (1960) 'Uncertainty in medical prognosis, clinical and functional', *American Journal of Sociology* 66: 41–7.

Davis, F. (1961) 'Deviance disavowal. The management of strained interaction by the visually handicapped', *Social Problems* 9: 120–32.

Davis, F. (1963) *Passage through Crisis: Polio Victims and their Families*, Indianapolis, Ind: Bobbs-Merrill.

Davis, M. Z. (1973) *Living with Multiple Sclerosis – A Social-Psychological Analysis*, Springfield, Ill: Charles C. Thomas.

Davoud, N. and Kettle, M. (1980) *MS and its Effect on Employment*, London: Multiple Sclerosis Society.

Detels, R., Clark, V. A., Valdiviezo, N. L., Visscher, B. R., Malmgren, R. M., and Dudley, J. P. (1982) 'Factors associated with a rapid course of multiple sclerosis', *Archives of Neurology* 39: 337–41.

DiMatteo, M. R. and Friedman, H. S. (1982) *Social Psychology and Medicine*, Cambridge, Mass: Oelgeschlager, Gunn & Hain.

Dunnell, K. and Cartwright, A. (1972) *Medicine Takers, Prescribers and Hoarders*, London: Routledge & Kegan Paul.

Duval, M. L. (1985) 'Psychosocial metaphors of physical distress among MS patients', *Social Science and Medicine* 19(6): 635–8.

Eisenberg, L. (1977) 'Disease and illness: distinctions between professional and popular ideas of sickness', *Culture, Medicine and Psychiatry* 1: 9–23.

Elian, M. and Dean, G. (1983) 'Need for and use of social and health services by multiple sclerosis patients in England and Wales', *Lancet* 14 May: 1,091–3.

Elian, M. and Dean, G. (1985) 'To tell or not to tell: the diagnosis of multiple sclerosis', *Lancet* 6 July: 27–8.

Feigenson, J. S., Scheinberg, L., Catalano, M., Polkow, L., Mantegazza, P. M., Feigenson, W. D., and LaRocca, N. G. (1981) 'The cost-effectiveness of multiple sclerosis rehabilitation: a model', *Neurology (Ny)* 31: 1,316–22.

Fitzpatrick, R., Hinton, J., Newman, S., Scambler, G., and Thompson, J. (1984) *The Experience of Illness*, London: Tavistock.

Fowler, C. J. (1987) 'Bladder and sexual dysfunction in multiple sclerosis', in F. C. Rose and R. Jones (eds) *Multiple Sclerosis*, London: J. Libbey.

Frankel, D. (1984) 'Long-term care issue in multiple sclerosis', *Rehabilitation Literature* 45: 282–5.

Freal, J. E., Kraft, G. H., and Coryell, J. K. (1984) 'Symptomatic fatigue in multiple sclerosis', *Archives of Physical Medicine and Rehabilitation* 65: 135–8.

Freer, C. B. (1980) 'Self-care: a diary study', *Medical Care* 18: 853–61.

Gale, J. and Marsden, P. (1985) 'Diagnosis: process not product', in M. Sheldon, J. Brook, and A. Rector (eds) *Decision Making in General Practice*, London: Macmillan.

Gallineck, A. and Kalinowsky, L. B. (1958) 'Psychiatric aspects of multiple sclerosis', *Diseases of the Nervous System* 19: 77–80.

Gay, D. and Dick, G. (1987) 'Is multiple sclerosis caused by an oral spirochaete? The evidence', in F. C. Rose and R. Jones (eds) *Multiple Sclerosis*, London: J. Libbey.

Gilbert, J. J. and Sadler, M. (1983) 'Unsuspected multiple sclerosis', *Archives of Neurology* 40: 533–6.

Glaser, B. G. (1972) 'Disclosure of terminal illness', in E. G. Jago (ed.) *Patients, Physicians and Illness*, Glencoe, Ill: Free Press.

Goffman, E. (1963) *Stigma*, Englewood Cliffs, NJ: Prentice-Hall.

Goodstein, R. K. and Ferrell, R. B. (1977) 'Multiple sclerosis – presenting as a depressive illness', *Diseases of the Nervous System* 38: 127–31.

Gorman, E., Rudd, A., and Ebers, G. C. (1984) 'Giving the diagnosis of multiple sclerosis', in C. M. Poser, D. W. Paty, L. C. Scheinberg, W. I. McDonald, and G. C. Ebers (eds) *The Diagnosis of Multiple Sclerosis*, New York: Thieme-Stratton.

Graham, J. (1981) *Multiple Sclerosis – A Self-Help Guide to its Management*, Wellingborough, Northants: Thorsons.

Grant, I. (1986) 'Neuropsychological and psychiatric disturbances in multiple sclerosis', in W. I. McDonald and D. H. Silberberg (eds) *Multiple Sclerosis*, London: Butterworths.

Helman, C. (1981) 'Disease versus illness in general practice', *Journal of the Royal College of General Practitioners* 31: 548–52.

Helman, C. (1984) *Culture, Health and Illness*, Bristol: Wright.

Hirsch, E. A. (1977) *Starting Over: The Autobiographical Account of a Psychologist's Experience with Multiple Sclerosis*, North Quincy, Mass: Christopher Publishing House.

James, P. B. (1982) 'Evidence for sub-acute fat embolism as the cause of multiple sclerosis', *Lancet*: 380–5.

James, P. B. (1987) 'The scientific basis for hyperbaric oxygen therapy', in F. C. Rose and R. Jones (eds) *Multiple Sclerosis*, London: J. Libbey.

Johnson, G. S. and Johnson, R. H. (1977) 'Social services support for multiple sclerosis patients in the west of Scotland', *Lancet* 1: 31–4.

Katz, A. H. (1979) 'Self-help groups: some clarifications', *Social Science and Medicine* 13: 491–4.

Kent, H. (1985) *Yoga for the Disabled*, Wellingborough, Northants: Thorsons.

Kraft, G. H., Freal, J. E., Coryell, J. K., Hanan, C. L., and Chitnis, N. (1981) 'Multiple sclerosis: early prognostic guidelines', *Archives of Physical Medicine and Rehabilitation* 62: 54–8.

Kraft, G. H., Freal, J. E., and Coryell, J. K. (1986) 'Disability, disease duration, and rehabilitation service needs in multiple sclerosis: patient perspectives', *Arch. Phys. Med. Rehab.* 67: 164–8.

Kurtzke, J. F. (1980) 'Multiple sclerosis: an overview', in F. C. Rose (ed.) *Clinical Neuroepidemiology*, London: Pitman Medical.

Kurtzke, J. F. and Hyllested, K. (1979) 'Multiple sclerosis in the Faroe Islands: (1) clinical and epidemiological features', *Annals of Neurology* 5: 6–21.

Lange, L. S. (1987) 'Multiple sclerosis: the viral dimension', in F. C. Rose and R. Jones (eds) *Multiple Sclerosis*, London: J. Libbey.

LaRocca, N. G. (1984) 'Psychosocial factors in multiple sclerosis and the role of stress', in L. C. Scheinberg and C. S. Raine (eds) *Multiple Sclerosis: Experimental and Clinical Aspects*, Annals of the New York Academy of Sciences, vol. 436.

LaRocca, N. G. and Holland, N. J. (1982) 'Vocational adjustment in multiple sclerosis', *American Rehabilitation* November/December 9–13.

LaRocca, N. G., Kalb, R., Scheinberg, L. C., and Kendall, P. (1985) 'Factors associated with unemployment of patients with multiple sclerosis', *Journal of Chronic Diseases* 38: 203–10.

Leibowitz, U., Antonowsky, A., Katz, R., and Alter, M. (1967) 'Does pregnancy increase the risk of multiple sclerosis', *Journal of Neurology, Neurosurgery and Psychiatry* 30: 354–7.

Ley, P. (1977) 'Psychological studies of doctor–patient communication', in S. Rachman (ed.) *Contributions to Medical Psychology*, vol. 1, Oxford: Pergamon Press.

Lincoln, N. B. (1981) 'Discrepancies between capabilities and performance of activities of daily living in multiple sclerosis patients', *International Rehabilitation Medicine* 3: 84–8.

Locker, D. (1981) *Symptoms and Illness*, London: Tavistock.

Locker, D. (1983) *Disability and Disadvantage*, London: Tavistock.

McAlpine, D., Lumsden, C. E., and Acheson, E. D. (1972) *Multiple Sclerosis: A Reappraisal*, Edinburgh: Churchill Livingstone.

McEwen, J., Martini, C. J. M., and Wilkins, N. (1983) *Participation in Health*, London: Croom Helm.

McIntosh, J. (1977) *Communication and Awareness in a Cancer Ward*, London: Croom Helm.

Marsh, G. G., Ellison, G. W., and Strite, C. (1983) 'Psychosocial and rehabilitation approaches to multiple sclerosis', *Annual Review of Rehabilitation*: 242–67.

Matson, R. R. and Brooks, N. A. (1977) 'Adjusting to multiple sclerosis – an exploratory study', *Social Science and Medicine* 11: 245–50.

Matthews, W. B. (1985) 'Clinical aspects', in W. B. Matthews, E. D. Acheson, J. R. Batchelor, and R. O. Weller, *McAlpine's Multiple Sclerosis*, Edinburgh: Churchill Livingstone.

Matthews, W. B., Acheson, E. D., Batchelor, J. R., and Weller, R. O. (1985) *McAlpine's Multiple Sclerosis*, Edinburgh: Churchill Livingstone.

Maybury, C. P. and Brewin, C. R. (1984) 'Social relationships, knowledge and adjustment to multiple sclerosis', *Journal of Neurology, Neurosurgery and Psychiatry* 47: 372–6.

Mayer, J. (1981) 'Geographic clues about multiple sclerosis', *Annals of the Association of American Geographers* 71: 28–39.

Mechanic, D. (1978) *Medical Sociology*, London: Collier-Macmillan.

Miles, A. (1979) 'Some psycho-social consequences of multiple sclerosis: problems of social interaction and group identity', *British Journal of Medical Psychology* 52: 321–31.

Miller, D. H., Ormerod, I. E. C., du Boulay, G. H., McDonald, W. I., Rudge, P., Kendall, B. E., Moseley, I. F., Johnson, G., Halliday, A. M., Scarivilla, F., Tofts, P. S., and Zilkha, K. J. (1987) 'A summary of the present contribution of magnetic resonance imaging to diagnosis and understanding of multiple sclerosis', in F. C. Rose and R. Jones (eds) *Multiple Sclerosis*, London: J. Libbey.

Mishler, E. G. (1981) *The Social Context of Health, Illness and Patient Care*, Cambridge: Cambridge University Press.

Monks, J. (1986) *Doing Justice to MS Symptoms*, general report no. 5, Brunel–ARMS Research Unit, Department of Human Sciences, Brunel, University of West London.

Morrell, D. C. and Wales, C. J. (1976) 'Symptoms perceived and recorded by patients', *Journal of Royal College of General Practitioners* 26: 398–403.

Murrell, T. G. C., O'Donoghue, P. J., and Ellis, T. (1986) 'A review of the sheep–multiple sclerosis connection', *Medical Hypotheses*, 19: 27–39.

National Childbirth Trust (1984) *The Emotions and Experiences of Disabled Mothers*, London: National Childbirth Trust.

Nicholas, J. (1982) 'Physiotherapy for multiple sclerosis', *Physiotherapy* 68: 144–6.

Novack, D., Plumer, R., Smith, R., Octihill, H., Morrow, G., and Bennett, J. (1979) 'Changes in physicians' attitudes towards telling the cancer patient', *Journal of the American Medical Association* 247: 897.

O'Brien, B. (1987) *Multiple Sclerosis*, London: Office of Health Economics.

Oken, D. (1961) 'What to tell cancer patients', *Journal of the American Medical Association* 175: 1,120.

Ormerod, I. E. C., McDonald, W. I., du Boulay, E. P. G. H., Kendall, B. E., Mosley, I. F., Halliday, A. M., Kakigi, R., Kirss, A., and Parringer, E. (1986) 'Disseminated lesions at presentation in patients with optic neuritis', *Journal of Neurosurgery and Psychiatry* 49: 124–7.

Parsons, T. (1952) *The Social System*, Glencoe, Ill: Free Press.

Paty, D. W. and Poser, C. (1984) 'Clinical signs and symptoms of multiple sclerosis', in D. Paty, W. I. McDonald, L. C. Scheinberg, and G. C. Ebers, *The Diagnosis of Multiple Sclerosis*, New York: Thieme-Stratton.

Peyser, J. M., Edwards, K. R., and Poser, C. M. (1980) 'Psychological profiles in patients with multiple sclerosis', *Archives of Neurology* 37: 437–40.

Pollock, K. (1984) *Mind and Matter*, PhD thesis, University of Cambridge.

Poser, C. M. (1984) 'Taxonomy and diagnostic parameters in multiple sclerosis', in L. C. Scheinberg and C. S. Raine (eds) *Multiple*

Sclerosis: Experimental and Clinical Aspects, Annals of the New York Academy of Sciences, vol. 436.

Poser, C. M. (1986) 'Pathogenesis of multiple sclerosis', *Acta Neurologica Pathologica* (Berlin): 1–10.

Poser, C. M., Paty, D. W., Scheinberg, L. C., McDonald, W. I., Davis, F. A., Ebers, G. C., Johnson, K. P., Sibley, W. A., Silberberg, D. H., and Tourtellote, W. W. (1983) 'New diagnostic criteria for multiple sclerosis: guidelines for research protocols', *Annals of Neurology* 13: 227–31.

Poser, S., Bauer, H. J., Ritter, G., Friedrich, H., Beland, H., and Denecke, P. (1981) 'Rehabilitation for patients with multiple sclerosis?' *Journal of Neurology* 224: 283–90.

Power, P. W. (1985) 'Family coping behaviours in chronic illness: a rehabilitation perspective', *Rehabilitation Literature* 46: 78–83.

Radford, I. and Trew, K. (1987) *Action for MS Care*, Action MS, The Inns, Saintfield Road, Belfast, N. Ireland.

Robinson, D. and Henry, S. (1977) *Self-Help and Health*, London: Martin Robertson.

Robinson, I. (1983) *Discovering the Diagnosis of MS*, general report no, 3, Brunel–ARMS Research Unit, Department of Human Sciences, Brunel, University of West London.

Robinson, I. (1986) 'Communicating the diagnosis of multiple sclerosis', paper presented to the Royal Society of Medicine Forum on Medical Communication.

Robinson, I. (1987a) 'Productive partnership? The profession and the patient in the management of multiple sclerosis', in F. C. Rose and R. Jones (eds) *Multiple Sclerosis*, London: J. Libbey.

Robinson, I. (1987b) 'Analysing the structure of 23 clinical trials in multiple sclerosis', *Neuroepidemiology* 6: 46–76.

Robinson, I. (1988) 'Reconstructing lives: Living with multiple sclerosis', in R. Anderson and M. Bury (eds) *Living with Chronic Disease*, London: Hyman Unwin.

Robinson, I., Bakes, C., and Lawson, A. (1983) *Questioning the Facts: The Sex Ratio in Multiple Sclerosis*, academic working paper, Brunel–ARMS Research Unit, Department of Human Sciences, Brunel, University of West London.

Robinson, I., Lawson, A., and Bakes, C. (1983) *MS People: A Demographic Profile*, general report no. 2, Brunel–ARMS Research Unit, Department of Human Sciences, Brunel, University of West London.

Robinson, I., Lawson, A., and Wynne, A. (1983) *Talking About MS*, general report no. 1, Brunel–ARMS Research Unit, Department of Human Sciences, Brunel, University of West London.

Rose, F. C. and Jones, R. (eds) (1987) *Multiple Sclerosis: Immunological, Diagnostic and Therapeutic Aspects*, London: J. Libbey.

Rosengren, W. R. (1980) *The Sociology of Medicine*, New York: Harper & Row.

Sainsbury, S. (1970) *Registered as Disabled*, occasional papers in social administration no. 35, London: G. Bell.

Scambler, G. (1984) 'Perceiving and coping with stigmatising illness', in R. Fitzpatrick, J. Hinton, S. Newman, G. Scambler, and J. Thompson, *The Experience of Illness*, London: Tavistock.

Scheinberg, L. C. ((1979) 'Studies in the long-term psychosocial problems of patients with multiple sclerosis', *International Journal of Rehabilitation Research* 2: 540–2.

Scheinberg, L. C. and Raine, C. S. (eds) (1984) *Multiple Sclerosis: Experimental and Clinical Aspects*, Annals of the New York Academy of Sciences, vol. 436.

Scheinberg, L. C., Holland, N. J., Kirschenbaum, M., Oaklander, A., and Geronemus, D. F. (1981) 'Comprehensive long-term care of patients with multiple sclerosis', *Neurology (Ny)* 31: 1,121–3.

Scheinberg, L. C., Kalb, R. C., LaRocca, N. G., Geisser, B. S., Slater, R. J., and Poser, C. M. (1984) 'The doctor–patient relationship in multiple sclerosis', in C. M. Poser, D. W. Paty, L. C. Scheinberg, W. I. McDonald, and G. C. Ebers, *The Diagnosis of Multiple Sclerosis*, New York: Thieme-Stratton.

Schiffer, R. B., Rudick, R. A,, and Herndon, R. M. (1983) 'Psychologic aspects of multiple sclerosis', *New York State Journal of Medicine* 83: 312–16.

Schumacher, G. A., Beebe, G. W., Kibler, R. F., Kurland, L. T., Kurtzke, J. F., McDowell, F., Nagler, B., Sibley, W. A., Tourtellotte, W. W., and Willmon, T. L. (1965) 'Problems of experimentals trials of therapy in multiple sclerosis', *Annals of the New York Academy of Sciences,* vol. 122: 552–68.

Simons, A. (ed.) (1984a) *Multiple Sclerosis: Psychological and Social Aspects*, London: Heinemann Medical.

Simons, A. (1984b) 'Problems of providing support for people with multiple sclerosis and their families', in A. Simons (ed.) *Multiple Sclerosis: Psychological and Social Aspects*, London: Heinemann Medical.

Simons, A. (1984c) 'Perceptions of health care', in A. Simons (ed.) *Multiple Sclerosis: Psychological and Social Aspects*, London: Heinemann Medical.

Slater, R. J., LaRocca, N. G., and Scheinberg, L. C. (1984) 'Development and testing of a minimal record of disability in Multiple Sclerosis', *Annals of the New York Academy of Sciences,* vol. 436: 453–468.

Smith, C. R. and Scheinberg, L. C. (1985) 'Clinical features of multiple sclerosis', *Seminars in Neurology* 5(2): 85–93.

Spielman, R. S. and Nathanson, N. (1982) 'The genetics of susceptibility to multiple sclerosis', *Epidemilogic Reviews* 4: 45–65.

Stewart, D. C. and Sullivan, T. J. (1982) 'Illness behaviour and the sick role: the case of multiple sclerosis', *Social Science and Medicine* 16: 1,397–1,404.

Strauss, A., Corbin, J., Sagerhaugh, S., Glaser, B. G., Maines, D.,

Suczek, B., and Wiener, C. L. (1984) *Chronic Illness and the Quality of Life* (2nd edn), Chicago, Ill: Mosby.

Suchman, E. (1965) 'Stages of illness and medical care', *Journal of Health and Social Behaviour* 6: 114–28.

Swingler, R. J. and Compston, D. A. S. (1986) 'The distribution of multiple sclerosis in the United Kingdom', *Journal of Neurology: Neurosurgery and Psychiatry* 49: 115–24.

Tuckett, D., Boulton, M., Olson, C., and Williams, A. (1985) *Meetings between Experts*, London: Tavistock.

Vanderplate, C. (1984) 'Psychological aspects of multiple sclerosis, and its treatment: towards a biopsychosocial perspective', *Health Psychology* 3: 253–72.

Wadsworth, M. E. J., Butterfield, W. H., and Blaney, R. (1971) *Health and Sickness: The Choice of Treatment*, London: Tavistock.

Walton, J. N. (1977) *Brain's Diseases of the Nervous System* (8th edn), Oxford: Oxford University Press.

Weller, R. O. (1985) 'Pathology of multiple sclerosis', in W. B. Matthews, E. D. Acheson, J. R. Batchelor, and R. O. Weller, *McAlpine's Multiple Sclerosis*, Edinburgh: Churchill Livingstone.

Whitlock, A. (1984) 'Emotional disorder in multiple sclerosis', in A. Simons (ed.) *Multiple Sclerosis: Psychological and Social Aspects*, London: Heinemann Medical.

Whitlock, F. A. and Siskind, D. M. M. (1980) 'Depression as a major symptom of multiple sclerosis', *Journal of Neurology, Neurosurgery, and Psychiatry* 43: 861–5.

Worthington, J. A., DeSouza, L. H., Forti, A., Jones, R., Modarres-Sadeghi, H., and Blaney, A. (1987) 'A double-blind controlled cross-over trial investigating the efficacy of hyperbaric oxygen in patients with multiple sclerosis', in F. C. Rose and R. Jones (eds) *Multiple Sclerosis*, London: J. Libbey.

Wright, B. A. (1983) *Physical Disability: A Psychosocial Approach* (2nd edn), New York: Harper & Row.

Zola, I. (1973) 'Pathways to the doctor: from person to patient', *Social Science and Medicine* 7: 677–88.

Index

Acheson, E. D., 3
ACTH, 12, 22, 27, 32, 83–4, 87–9
Alaszewski, A., 95
Alter, M., 7, 9, 10, 12
'alternative' therapies, 23, 86–92
Anderson, J. A. D., 87
animals (associated with MS), 9
ARMS (Action for Research into
    Multiple Sclerosis), 95, 103,
    120–4, 126, 128, 135

Bakes, C., 8, 61
Baretz, R. M., 46
Beck, R. P., 43
Birrer, C., 42
Blaxter, M., 36, 38, 58, 61, 106,
    110–12
body (relationship with), 41–5
Briggs, A., 56, 67, 112
Brooks, N. A., 32–3, 35–6, 46
Brown, S., 45
Burnfield, A., 41, 50, 57, 81, 90,
    118, 123, 132
Bury, M., 112

Campling, J., 43, 47
Cartright, A., 14
Cassell, E. J., 42
cerebro-spinal fluid, 4
charitable organizations, 114–24
Charmaz, K., 131, 136
children, 59, 60, 68–73
Cleeland, C. S., 46

Compston, A., 6
computerized tomography (CT), 4
Cornwell, J., 131
Coryell, J. K., 106
Cottrell, S. S., 45
Cunningham, D. J., 18, 21, 30,
    51–2, 56, 57, 62–3, 65, 67,
    72–3, 76, 114

Davis, F., 22, 51, 53
Davis, M. Z., 114
Davis, T. K., 45
Davoud, N., 73–4
Dean, G., 24–5, 26, 27, 101–3,
    106–7, 111, 112
dependence, 44, 62–8
depression, 20, 45–8
deviance disavowal, 53
DHSS, 109–10
diagnosis: 2–3; criteria, 3;
    discovery of, 24–32; quest for,
    21–4; reactions to, 29–36, see
    also strategies; techniques,
    4–5, 22
diet, 10, 80, 87–8, 92–5, 121–2,
    128
DiMatteo, M. R., 32
divorce, 61–2
doctor–patient relationships,
    18–27, 81–6, 101–5
drug therapies, 12, 82–3, see also
    ACTH
Dunnell, K., 14

Ebers, G. C., 58
Edwards, K. R., 46–7
Elian, M., 24–5, 26, 27, 101–3, 106–7, 111, 112
Ellison, G. W., 45, 135
employment, 39–40, 67, 73–77, 110–11
euphoria, 45–8
exercise, 88, 92, 93, 96–7, 128
eyesight, 4–5, 16, 51–2

family, 57, 66–7, 106, 112–13, 125, 134–5
Faroe Islands, 9
fat embolism, 10–11
Ferrell, R. B., 46
Freal, J. E., 106
Friedman, H. S., 32
friends, 50, 57, 61, 112–14, 125

Gale, J., 19, 21
Gallineck, A., 46
genetic factors, 11
Gerson therapy, 94
Gilbert, J. J., 4
Glaser, B. G., 25
Goffman, E., 51, 52
Goodstein, R. K., 46
Gorman, E., 58
GP, *see* doctor
Graham, Judy, 87, 89
Grant, I., 99

Harshe, M., 10
HBO (hyperbaric oxygen), 88, 121–2, 126, 128–9
Helman, C., 78–9, 92
Henry, S., 114–15
Herndon, R. M., 47
Hirsch, E. A., 37–8
Holland, N. J., 73
home (going into a), 64
Hopper, C. L., 46
Hyllested, K., 9

identity spread, 57
imaging techniques, 4, 126
immunological system, 10
incontinence, 38, 43–4

institutional solution, 64
International Federation of Multiple Sclerosis Societies, 117

James, P. B., 10–11

Kalinowsky, L. B., 46
Katz, A. H., 116
Kettle, M., 73–4
Kraft, G. H., 38, 106
Kurtzke, J. F., 7, 9

Lancet, 24
LaRocca, N. G., 73–4
Lawson, A., 8, 44, 61, 76
Leibowitz, U., 7, 69
limping, 17, 51
Lincoln, N. B., 65
Locker, D., 66
Lumsden, C. E., 3

McAlpine, D., 3
McDougall, Roger, 94
McEwen, J., 86–7, 114–15
marriages, 58–61
Marsden, P., 19, 21
Marsh, G. G., 45, 135
Martini, C. J. M., 86–7, 114–15
Matson, R. R., 32–3, 35–6, 46
Matthews, C. G., 46
Matthews, W. B., 6, 16, 69, 92
Mayer, J., 8
measles virus, 10, 80
Mechanic, D., 14, 26
media (role of), 115
Medical Research Advisory Committee, 118
Medical Research Council, 127
Miles, A., 51, 53–7, 116
Miller, D. H., 4
Mishler, E. G., 29
Monks, J., 41
multiple sclerosis (MS): cause, 8–11; course of, 6; description, 1–2; diagnosis, *see* diagnosis; distribution, 7–8; employment, *see* employment; explanations for, 78–81; information, 26, 83,

85, 104, 129–31; investigations, 2; management, 11–13, 32–6, 78–81, 97–100; medical support, 101–5; nature, 13; onset, 14–21; pathology, 4–5; 'personality type', 45–8; prognosis, 6; relationships, 57–61, 134–5; research, 118, 121, 126; social context, 50–7, 77; social roles, 61–8; societies, 117–24; strategies, *see* strategies; supernatural beliefs, 79, 98, 131–4; support agencies, 105–11; symptoms, *see* symptoms; variability, 2, 14, 38
Multiple Sclerosis Society, 117–19, 121–4, 126
Murrell, T. G. C., 9

Nathanson, N., 11
National Childbirth Trust, 69
Novack, D., 25
nuclear magnetic resonance (NMR), 4, 126
nutrition, *see* diet

O'Brien, B., 110
Oken, D., 25
Oliver, J., 56, 67, 112
optic neuritis, 4, 16
Ormerod, I. E. C., 4

personality types, 45–8
Peyser, J. M., 46–7
physiotherapy, 95–6, 108, 121
plaques, sclerotic, 4
plateaux, 89
Pollock, K., 33
Poser, C. M., 2, 3, 5, 11, 46–7, 103
Poser, S., 144
Power, P. W., 66–7
prednisone, 12
pregnancy, 69–70

Radford, I., 24, 26, 65, 101, 103, 106, 111, 112
religious beliefs, 79, 98, 131–4
Robinson, D., 114–15

Robinson, I., 8, 24, 26, 30, 32, 34, 44, 57, 61, 65, 76, 80, 85, 103, 127
Rosengren, W. R., 81
Rudd, A., 58
Rudick, R. A., 47

Sadler, M., 4
Sainsbury, S., 58
Scambler, G., 29–30
Scheinberg, L. C., 24, 25, 26
Schiffer, R. B., 47
Schumacher, G. A., 2, 3, 5
self-care, 86–92
self-help groups, 114
self-image, 39, 45–8, 76
sexuality, 43, 63
Simons, A., 95
Siskind, D. M. M., 46
social services, 108
Speer, J., 8
Spielman, R. S., 11
Stephenson, G. R., 46
steroids, *see* drug therapies
Stewart, D. C., 14, 15, 18, 19, 21, 22, 23, 29, 36
strategies: accepting, 33–4, 35, 48, 135–6; alternative medical, 86–91; coping, 33–6, 66, 135–6; denial, 32–3, 35, 48; dietary, 94; disassociation, 51, 56–7; fighting, 33–6, 48, 136; integration, 33–4, 35; mental control, 98–9; normalization, 51, 53–6; passing, 51–3; research, 83, 129–31
Strauss, A., 37, 39, 40, 49, 54, 57, 61, 65
Strite, C., 45, 135
Suchman, E., 15
Sullivan, T. J., 14, 15, 18, 19, 21, 22, 23, 29, 36
symptoms: describing, 41; interpreting, 5–6; multiplicity, 2, 14, 20, 38; pathological signs, 4–5; recognizing, 14–21; *see also* eyesight, fatigue, incontinence

Trew, K., 24, 26, 65, 101, 103, 106, 111, 112
Tuckett, D., 130

uncertainty, 36–40
unemployment, *see* employment
urinary problems, *see* incontinence

Vanderplate, C., 33
visually evoked potentials (VEP), 5

Walton, J. N., 1
Warren, E. G., 43
wheelchairs, 37, 44–5, 55, 106, 107, 109–10
Whitlock, A., 46
Whitlock, F. A., 46
Whitman, P., 43
Wilkins, N., 86–7, 114–15
Wilson, S. A., 45
work, *see* employment
Wright, B. A., 36–7, 38, 39, 42, 62, 135–6
Wynne, A., 44, 76

Yamoor, M., 10
yoga, 88, 96–7

Zola, I., 91